The Complete

DIVERTICULITIS

Diet Cookbook

1500

Days of Nourishing Recipes for Gut Wellness. Includes a 30-Day Meal Plan through an essential Tri-Phase Nutrition Guide For Lasting Digestive Health

Patti Blake

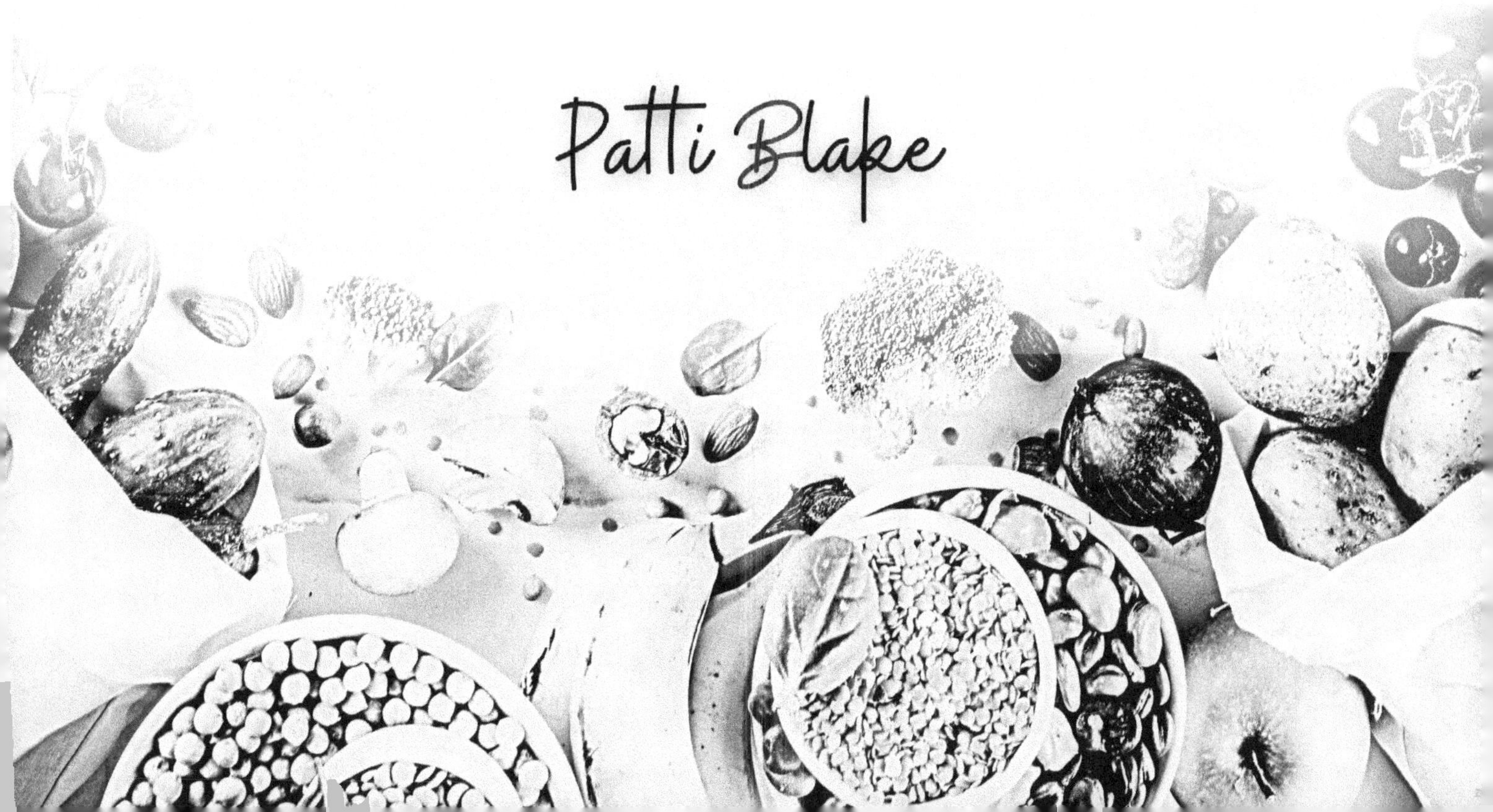

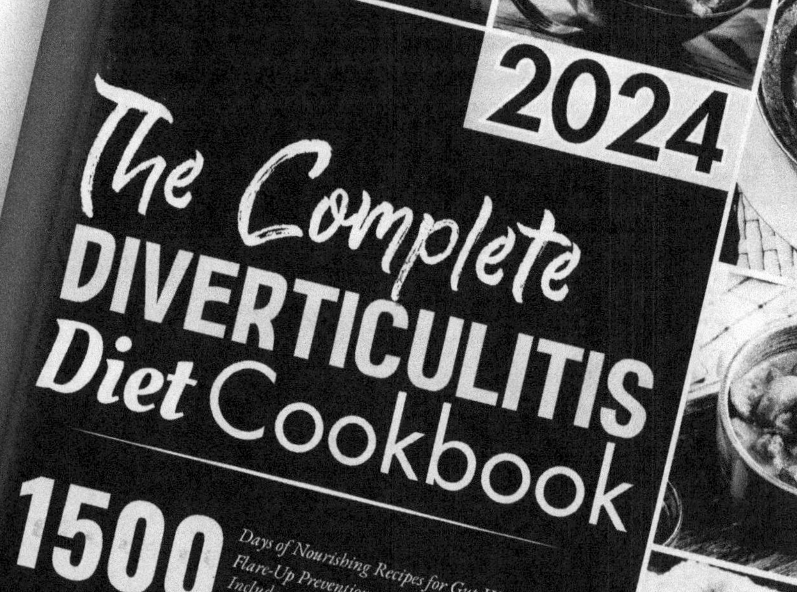
2024
The Complete
DIVERTICULITIS
Diet Cookbook
1500
Days of Nourishing Recipes for Gut Wellness and Flare-Up Prevention.
Includes a 30-Day Meal Plan through an essential Tri-Phase Nutrition Guide For Lasting Digestive Health.
30 DAYS MEAL PLAN
3 BONUSES INCLUDED
Patti Blake

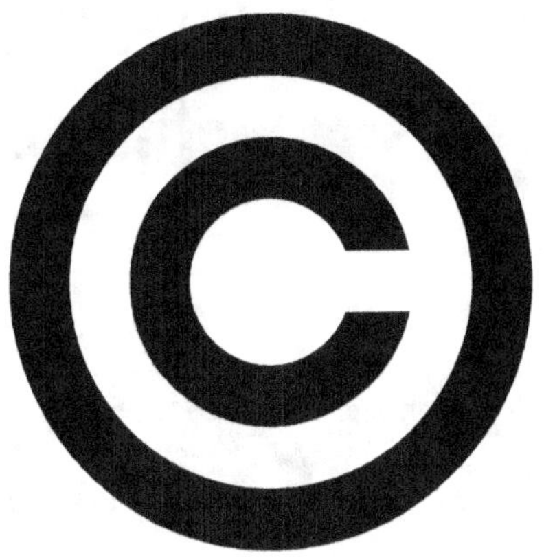

Copyright © 2024 by Patti Blake

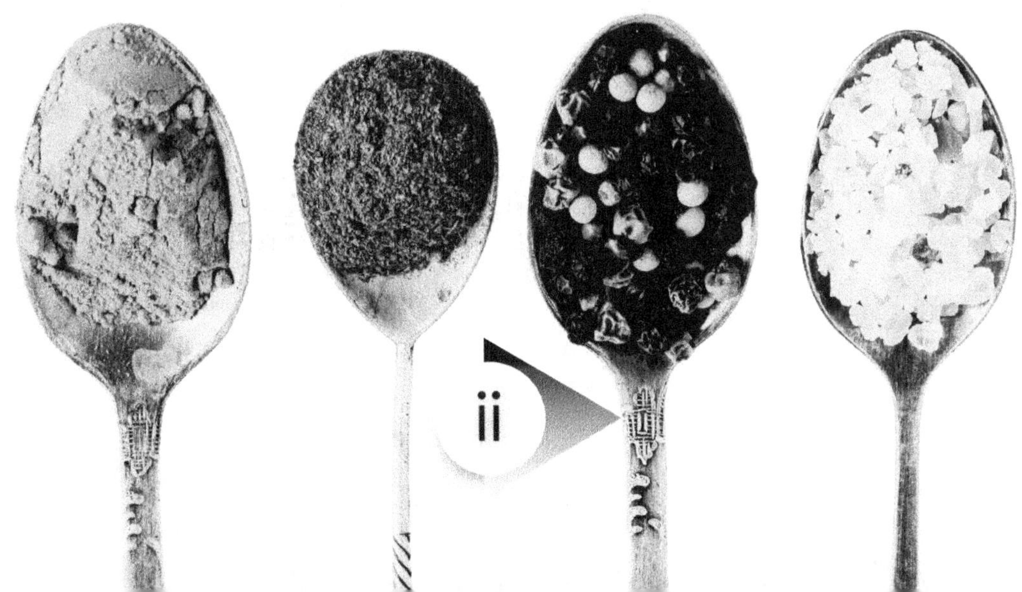

Scan the QR code at the end of the book to get your bonus!

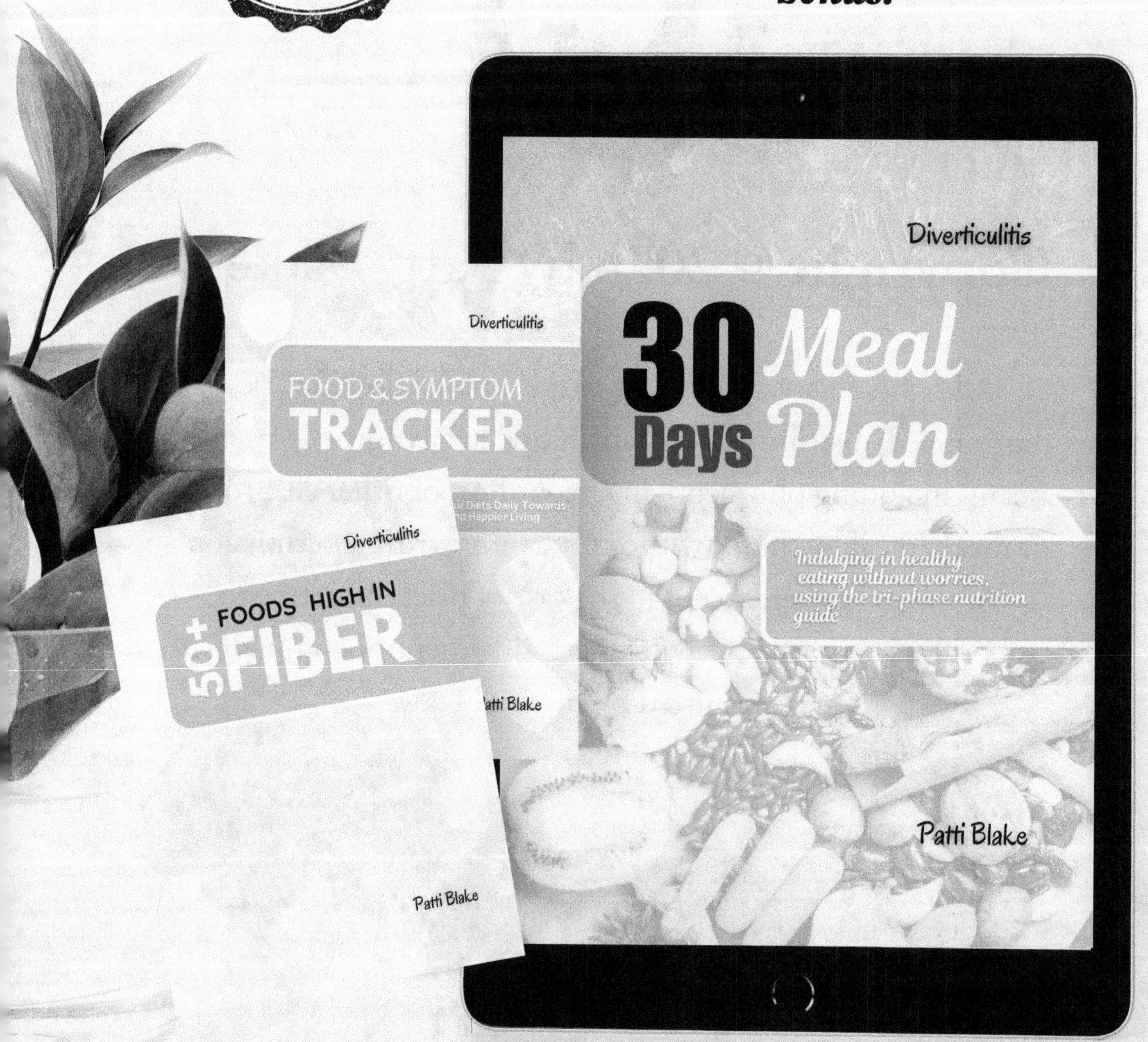

Table of contents

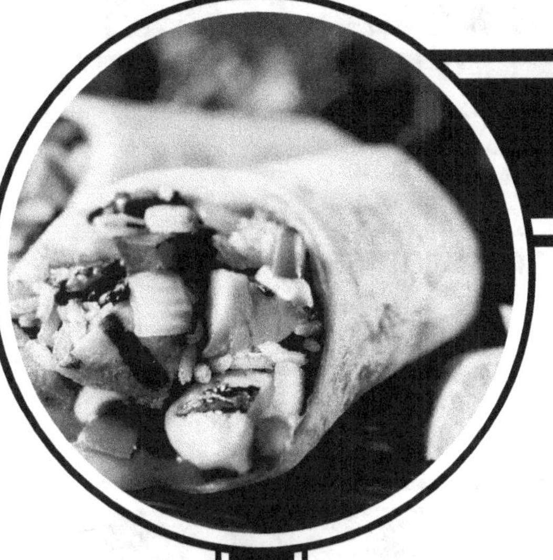

Introduction

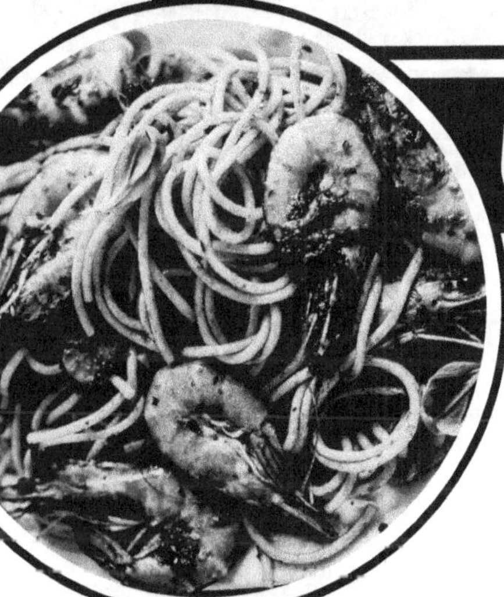

Understanding Diverticulitis

- Overview of Diverticulitis
- Types of Diverticulitis
- Causes and Risk Factors
- Symptoms and Diagnosis

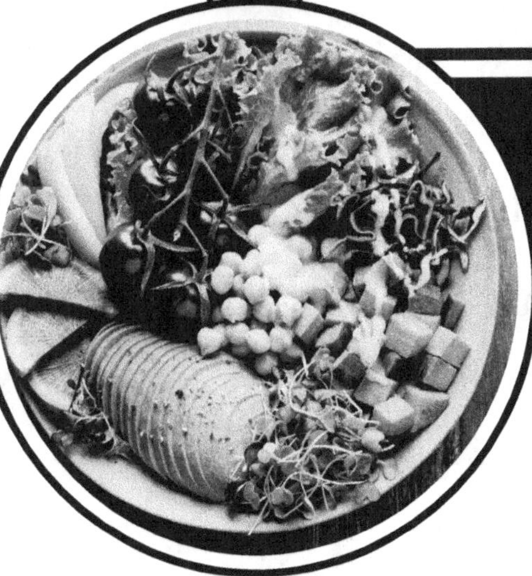

Importance of Nutrition in Diverticulitis Management

- Role of Diet in Preventing and Managing Diverticulitis
- Three Stages of Nutrition Guide
- Benefits of Following a Structured Diet Plan
- Natural Healing And Supplements

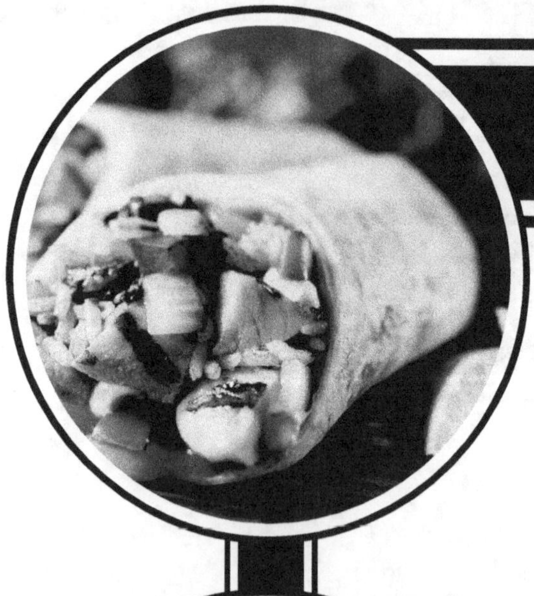

- Stage 1: Acute Diverticulitis Recovery
- Stage 2: Healing and Stabilization
- Stage 3: Maintenance and Prevention

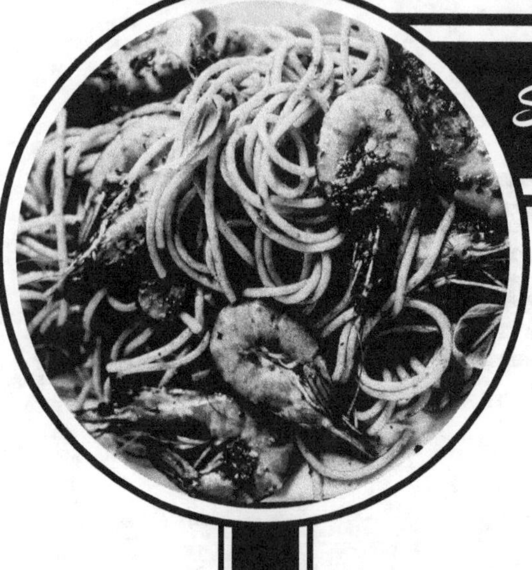

Stage 1: Acute Diverticulitis Recovery recipe

Breakfast Recipes

1. Banana Smoothie
2. Vegetable Broth
3. Applesauce
4. Greek Yogurt with Honey
5. Rice Porridge
6. Scrambled Eggs
7. Oatmeal Porridge
8. Cream of Wheat

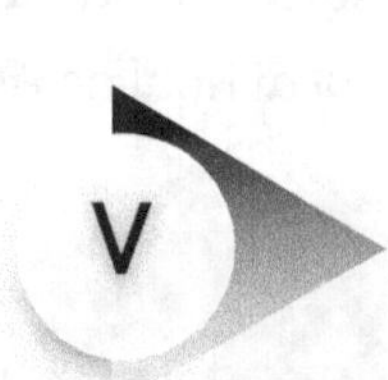

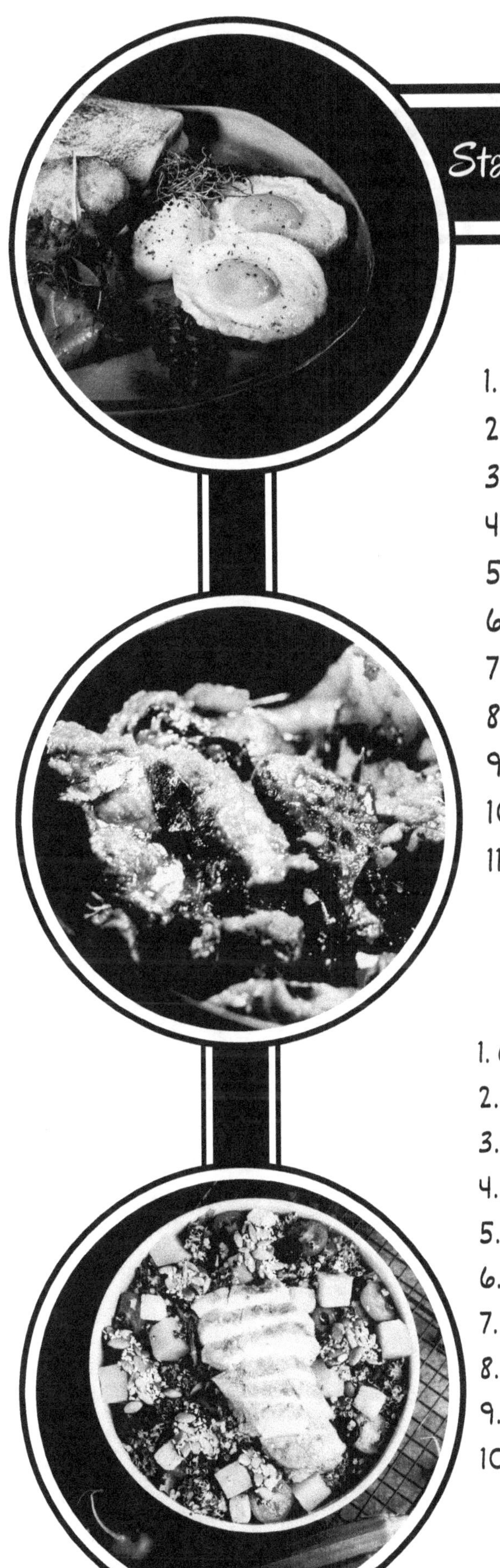

Lunch Recipes

1. Clear Chicken Broth
2. Herbal Tea with Lemon
3. Clear Vegetable Broth with Steamed Carrots
4. Fruit Gelatin Cups
5. Apple Juice
6. Green tea with honey
7. Citrus Gelatin mold
8. Mashed Butternut Squash
9. Steamed White Fish
10. Boiled Eggs with Steamed Spinach
11. Mashed Butternut Squash

Dinner Recipes

1. Clear Vegetable Broth with Steamed Green Beans
2. Herbal Infusion with Soft Tofu
3. Mashed Pumpkin with Rice
4. Clear Beef Consommé with Soft Noodles
5. Jellied Cranberry Sauce with Greek Yogurt
6. Apple Cider with Boiled Potatoes
7. Lemon Infused Water with Scrambled Eggs
8. Soft Polenta with Cooked Carrots
9. Pear Juice with Baked Chicken Breast
10. Pineapple Gelatin Cups with Cottage Cheese

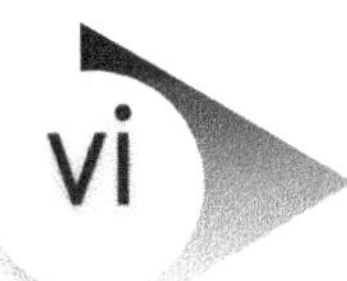

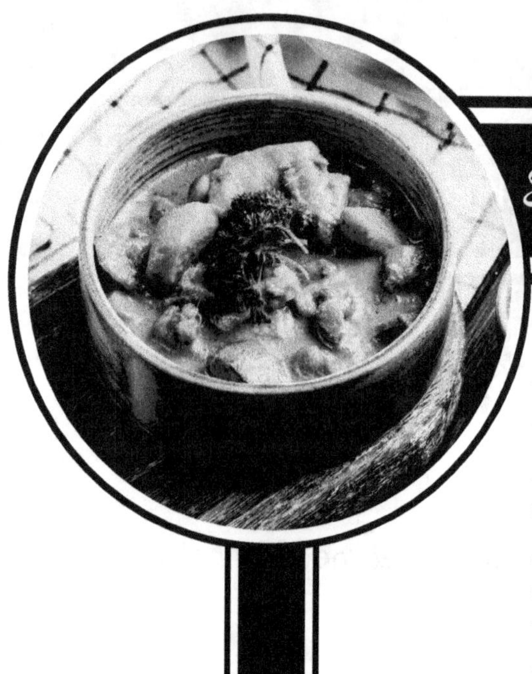

Breakfast Recipes

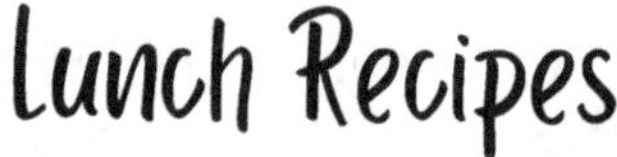

Lunch Recipes

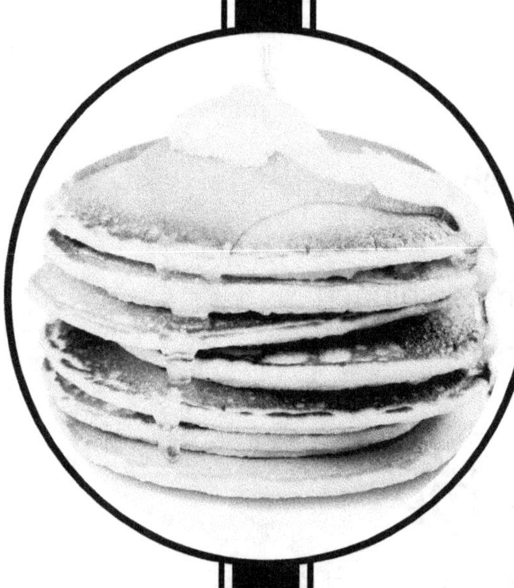

Dinner Recipes

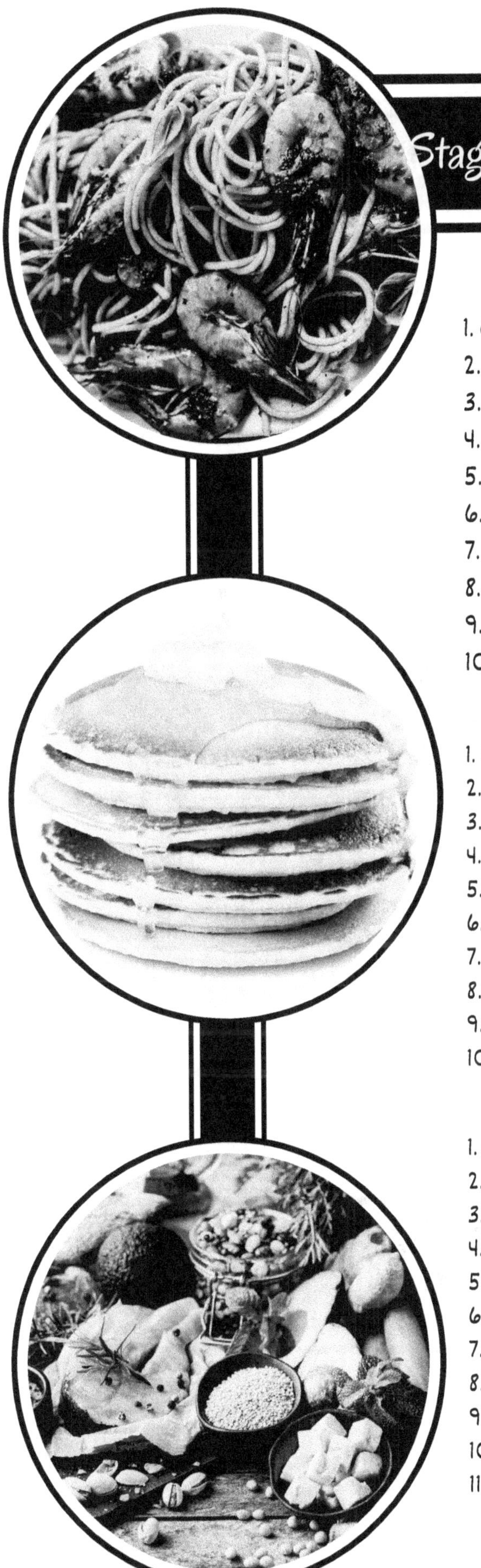

Breakfast Recipes

1. Chia Seed Breakfast Bowl
2. Sweet Potato Hash with Poached Eggs
3. Buckwheat Pancakes with Blueberry Compote
4. Veggie Omelette
5. Greek Yogurt Parfait with Almond Granola
6. Spinach and Feta Breakfast Quesadilla
7. Overnight Oats with Peanut Butter and Banana
8. Smoked Salmon Breakfast Bagel
9. Quinoa Breakfast Porridge
10. Avocado Toast with Poached Eggs

Lunch Recipes

1. Mediterranean Chickpea Salad
2. Grilled Veggie Wrap
3. Turkey and Avocado BLT
4. Quinoa and Black Bean Salad
5. Tuna Salad Stuffed Bell Peppers
6. Veggie and Hummus Plate
7. Chicken and Quinoa Bowl
8. Salmon Salad Lettuce Wraps
9. Lentil Soup with Whole Grain Bread
10. Veggie Sushi Rolls

Dinner Recipes

1. Lemon Garlic Salmon
2. Turkey Meatloaf with Mashed Cauliflower
3. Stuffed Acorn Squash
4. Mediterranean Chicken Skewers
5. Cauliflower Fried Rice
6. Spinach and Mushroom Stuffed Chicken
7. Baked Eggplant Rollatini
8. Lemon Herb Quinoa Pilaf
9. Roasted Vegetable Frittata
10. Eggplant Parmesan
11 Baked Cod with Herb Crust

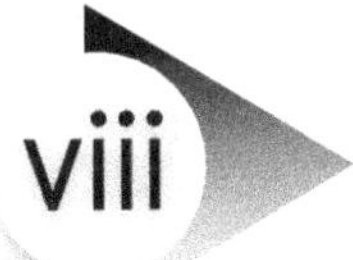

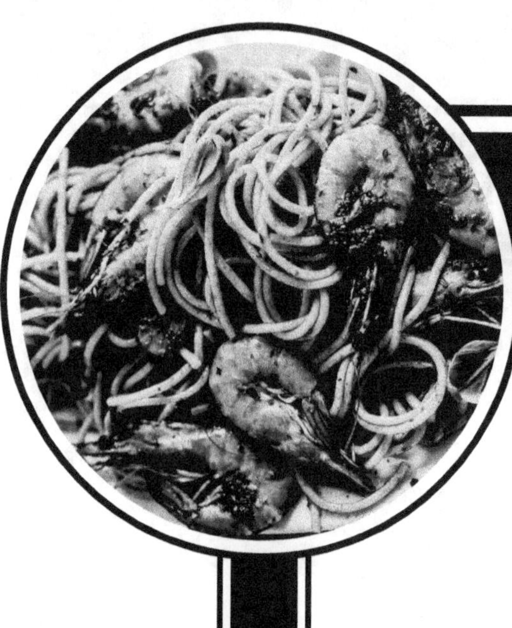

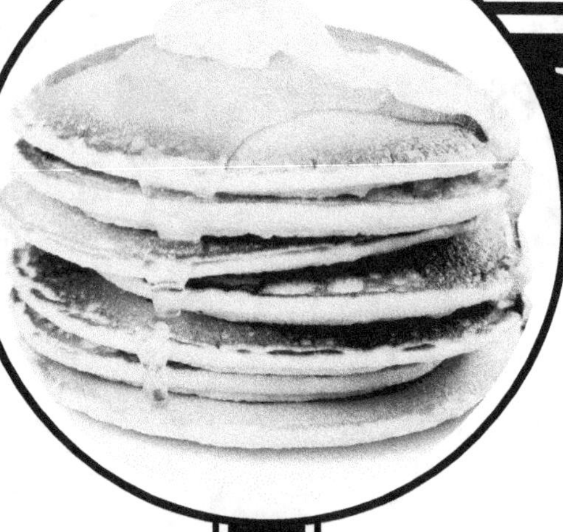

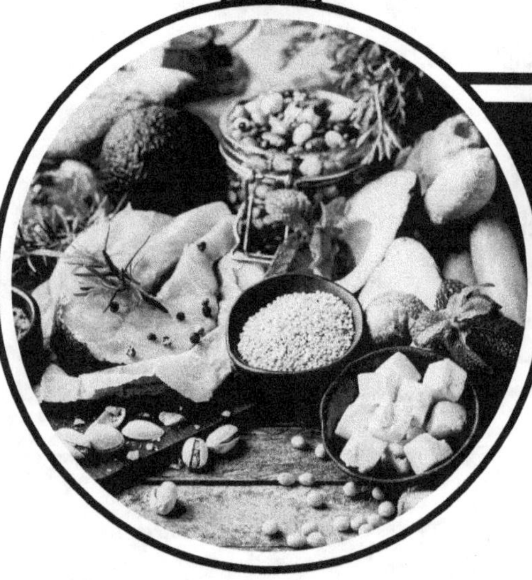

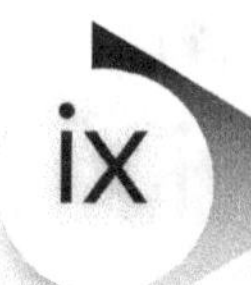

Introduction

Welcome to the Diverticulitis Diet Cookbook, where delicious recipes meet the science of managing a challenging condition. I'm thrilled to embark on this journey with you as we explore the crucial role nutrition plays in navigating diverticulitis

For many, the term "diverticulitis" can evoke a sense of uncertainty and even fear. It's a condition that affects millions of people worldwide, characterized by the formation of small pouches, called diverticula, in the lining of the digestive system, typically the colon. While the exact cause of diverticulitis remains elusive, several factors, including age, genetics, and lifestyle, may contribute to its development.

Living with diverticulitis can present various challenges, from managing symptoms during flare-ups to adopting long-term dietary changes to prevent recurrences. As someone passionate about the intersection of food and health, I understand the profound impact that diet can have on our well-being, particularly for individuals managing digestive conditions like diverticulitis.

In this cookbook, we'll embark on a journey together, guided by three essential principles: understanding, nourishment, and empowerment. We'll delve into the nuances of diverticulitis, exploring its causes, symptoms, and treatment options, empowering you with knowledge to make informed decisions about your health.

But knowledge alone isn't enough. We'll also dive into the practical aspects of managing diverticulitis through nutrition, providing you with a comprehensive guide to crafting delicious meals that support digestive health and overall well-being. From soothing soups to satisfying main dishes, each recipe is carefully crafted to prioritize ingredients that are gentle on the digestive system while still tantalizing your taste buds.

Beyond recipes, we'll explore strategies for success in various situations, from dining out with friends to navigating social gatherings. You'll find practical tips for meal planning, grocery shopping, and incorporating stress management techniques into your daily routine—because managing diverticulitis isn't just about what you eat; it's about how you live.

As we embark on this culinary journey together, remember that you're not alone. Whether you're newly diagnosed or a seasoned veteran in managing diverticulitis, this cookbook is designed to be your trusted companion, offering support, guidance, and, above all, delicious recipes to nourish both body and soul.

So let's roll up our sleeves, tie on our aprons, and dive into the flavorful world of diverticulitis-friendly cuisine. Together, we'll discover that eating well isn't just about managing a condition—it's about embracing a vibrant, fulfilling life.

Let's get cooking!

Chapter 1
Understanding Diverticulitis

Diverticulitis is a multifaceted gastrointestinal condition that demands attention to detail and a nuanced understanding of its various presentations. Let's delve deeper into the intricacies of this condition to shed light on its complexities.

Overview of Diverticulitis

Diverticulitis is marked by inflammation or infection within the diverticula, small pouches that protrude from the walls of the colon. While the condition can manifest in different forms, ranging from mild discomfort to severe complications, it's essential to grasp the nuances of each presentation.

Types of Diverticulitis

Diverticulitis can present in several distinct forms, each with its own set of characteristics and implications:

1. Uncomplicated Diverticulitis:

This is the most prevalent form, characterized by localized inflammation within a diverticulum. Symptoms typically include left lower quadrant abdominal pain, ranging from mild cramping to a dull ache. Constipation, bloating, and a low-grade fever may also occur. Treatment often involves conservative management, including a clear liquid diet followed by a gradual reintroduction of high-fiber foods. Pain medication and antibiotics may be prescribed depending on severity.

2. Acute Complicated Diverticulitis:

This presentation signifies a more significant inflammatory process, potentially involving complications such as abscess formation or perforation. Symptoms become more intense and persistent, often accompanied by fever, nausea, vomiting, and possibly blood in the stool. Treatment requires intravenous antibiotics, hospitalization, and sometimes surgical intervention to address complications.

3. Chronic Diverticulitis:

While not a distinct type, chronic diverticulitis represents a consequence of recurrent acute episodes. Symptoms may include recurrent abdominal pain, albeit often less severe than the initial attack, and changes in bowel habits like alternating constipation and diarrhea. Prevention of further flare-ups is key, with a focus on maintaining a high-fiber diet, hydration, stress management, and medications to regulate bowel movements and reduce inflammation. Surgery may be considered if conservative measures fail to control symptoms.

Causes and Risk Factors

Diverticulitis's precise etiology is unknown, although a number of variables are thought to be involved in its development. These include:

Low-Fiber Diet:

A diet low in fiber can lead to constipation and increased pressure within the colon, predisposing individuals to the formation of diverticula.

Aging:

The risk of diverticulitis increases with age, with the condition being more common in individuals over the age of 50.

Genetics:

There may be a genetic component to the development of diverticulitis, as individuals with a family history of the condition are at higher risk.

Lifestyle Factors:

Factors such as obesity, sedentary behavior, and smoking have been associated with an increased risk of diverticulitis.

Symptoms and Diagnosis

Diverticulitis symptoms can vary in severity and presentation, ranging from mild discomfort to more severe complications. Let's break down each symptom of diverticulitis

1. Abdominal Pain:

- This is a hallmark symptom of diverticulitis and is often localized to the lower left side of the abdomen.
- The pain may range from mild cramping to a more severe, constant ache.
- It can be exacerbated by movements such as walking or coughing and may persist for several days.

2. Bloating:

- Bloating refers to a feeling of fullness or tightness in the abdomen, often accompanied by a sensation of swelling or distention.
- It can contribute to discomfort and a sense of heaviness in the abdominal region.

3. Constipation:

- Constipation is referred to as irregular or uncomfortable bowel movements.
- It may be characterized by straining during bowel movements and a feeling of incomplete evacuation.
- Constipation can exacerbate abdominal pain and discomfort.

4. Low-Grade Fever:

- A low-grade fever refers to a slight increase in body temperature, typically ranging from 100.4°F (38°C) to 101°F (38.3°C).
- It may indicate the presence of inflammation or infection in the body, such as that seen in diverticulitis.

5. Nausea and Vomiting:

- Nausea refers to a sensation of queasiness or discomfort in the stomach, often accompanied by an urge to vomit.
- Vomiting is the forced ejection of stomach contents through the mouth.
- These symptoms may be triggered by abdominal pain and can contribute to dehydration and further discomfort.

6. Fever:

- Fever is a higher-than-normal body temperature, typically exceeding 100.4°F (38°C).
- It indicates the presence of inflammation or infection in the body and can be a sign of a more severe diverticulitis flare-up.

7. Blood in the Stool:

- Blood in the stool, known as hematochezia, may manifest as bright red or maroon-colored blood or as dark, tarry stools (melena).
- It can indicate bleeding within the digestive tract, which may occur as a complication of severe diverticulitis or other gastrointestinal conditions.

Chapter 2

Importance of Nutrition in Diverticulitis Management

Nutrition plays a pivotal role in managing diverticulitis, offering a powerful tool for both prevention and treatment. By understanding the impact of diet on digestive health and adopting a structured approach to nutrition, individuals can effectively manage symptoms, reduce the risk of flare-ups, and promote overall well-being.

Role of Diet in Preventing and Managing Diverticulitis:

Imagine your digestive system as a finely tuned machine, requiring the right fuel to function optimally. Diet plays a critical role in maintaining digestive health, particularly in the context of diverticulitis. A diet rich in fiber and hydration can help promote regular bowel movements, prevent constipation, and reduce pressure within the colon, thus decreasing the risk of diverticula formation and inflammation.

Furthermore, certain dietary factors, such as processed foods high in refined sugars and low in fiber, can exacerbate symptoms and increase the likelihood of diverticulitis flare-ups. By making informed choices about food intake, individuals can mitigate these risks and support their digestive health.

Three Stages of Nutrition Guide:

Navigating the dietary landscape of diverticulitis management can feel overwhelming, but fear not—there's a structured approach to guide you through the process. The Diverticulitis Diet Cookbook offers a three-stage nutrition guide designed to support individuals at different stages of their journey:

1. Acute Diverticulitis Recovery:

During this initial phase, when symptoms are acute and inflammation is present, the focus is on gentle, easily digestible foods that provide nourishment without exacerbating symptoms. A clear liquid diet may be recommended initially to allow the colon to rest and inflammation to subside. This stage gradually transitions to low-fiber foods as symptoms improve.

2. Healing and Stabilization:

As symptoms subside and inflammation resolves, the focus shifts to introducing high-fiber foods back into the diet to promote regular bowel movements and prevent future flare-ups. This stage emphasizes a balanced diet rich in fruits, vegetables, whole grains, and legumes, along with adequate hydration to support digestive health.

3. Maintenance and Prevention:

Once symptoms are under control, the emphasis is on maintaining a healthy diet and lifestyle to prevent recurrence of diverticulitis. This stage involves incorporating a variety of high-fiber foods into daily meals, staying hydrated, and practicing stress management techniques to support overall well-being.

Benefits of Following a Structured Diet Plan

Adopting a structured diet plan tailored to the specific needs of individuals with diverticulitis offers numerous benefits, including:

Symptom Management:

A well-planned diet can help alleviate symptoms such as abdominal pain, bloating, and irregular bowel movements, improving quality of life.

Prevention of Flare-Ups:

By avoiding trigger foods and incorporating dietary strategies to promote digestive health, individuals can reduce the risk of diverticulitis flare-ups and complications.

Improved Nutritional Status:

A balanced diet rich in fiber, vitamins, and minerals supports overall health and well-being, providing essential nutrients for optimal functioning of the body.

Long-Term Health:

By adopting healthy eating habits and lifestyle practices, individuals can promote long-term digestive health and reduce the risk of developing other chronic conditions associated with poor diet and lifestyle choices.

Natural Healing And Supplements

When it comes to managing diverticulitis, supplements and natural remedies can play a supportive role alongside dietary changes and medical treatments. Below are some of the major options to consider:

1. Probiotics:

Probiotic supplements contain beneficial bacteria that can help restore balance to the gut microbiome. They may reduce inflammation, improve digestion, and enhance immune function. Look for probiotic supplements containing strains such as Lactobacillus acidophilus, Bifidobacterium bifidum, and Lactobacillus plantarum.

2. Fiber supplements:

During the acute phase of diverticulitis, a low-fiber diet is often recommended to reduce irritation to the digestive tract. However, once symptoms subside, gradually increasing fiber intake is essential for long-term management. Fiber supplements such as psyllium husk or methylcellulose can help ensure an adequate intake of soluble fiber, which promotes regular bowel movements and supports gut health.

3. Digestive enzymes:

Digestive enzyme supplements can aid in the breakdown and absorption of nutrients, easing the burden on the digestive system. Enzymes like amylase, protease, and lipase can help improve digestion and reduce symptoms such as bloating, gas, and discomfort.

4. Fish oil:

Digestive enzyme supplements can aid in the breakdown and absorption of nutrients, easing the burden on the digestive system. Enzymes like amylase, protease, and lipase can help improve digestion and reduce symptoms such as bloating, gas, and discomfort.

5. Aloe vera:

Aloe vera has long been used for its soothing properties and may help alleviate inflammation and irritation in the digestive tract. Drinking aloe vera juice or taking aloe vera supplements may provide relief from symptoms such as abdominal pain and discomfort.

6. Marshmallow root:

Marshmallow root contains mucilage, a gel-like substance that coats and soothes the lining of the digestive tract. It may help alleviate symptoms of diverticulitis such as inflammation and irritation. Marshmallow root supplements are available in capsule or powder form.

7. Slippery elm:

Similar to marshmallow root, slippery elm contains mucilage and can help soothe inflammation in the digestive tract. It may also help relieve symptoms such as diarrhea and constipation. Slippery elm supplements are available in various forms, including capsules, powder, and lozenges.

8. Turmeric:

Curcumin, the active compound in turmeric, has potent anti-inflammatory and antioxidant properties. Incorporating turmeric supplements or adding turmeric powder to your diet may help reduce inflammation and promote gut health.

It's essential to consult with a healthcare professional before starting any new supplements or natural remedies, especially if you have underlying health conditions or are taking medications. They can provide personalized recommendations and ensure that the supplements you choose are safe and appropriate for your individual needs. Additionally, remember that supplements are meant to complement, not replace, a healthy diet and lifestyle.

Chapter 3
The Three Stage Nutrition Guide to diverticulitis

Stage 1: Acute Diverticulitis Recovery

Navigating the Acute Phase

Facing the acute phase of diverticulitis can be a daunting experience, but fear not—there's a roadmap to guide you through this challenging terrain. Let's explore the essential strategies for navigating the acute phase of diverticulitis recovery with confidence and ease.

Clear Liquid Diet: What to Eat and Avoid

During the acute phase of diverticulitis, when inflammation is at its peak and the digestive system is in distress, a clear liquid diet can provide much-needed relief. This diet consists of easily digestible liquids that provide hydration and essential nutrients without exacerbating symptoms. Here's what to include and avoid:

What to Eat:

- **Clear broths:** Chicken, vegetable, or beef broths are excellent options for providing nourishment and hydration.
- **Herbal teas:** Non-caffeinated herbal teas, such as chamomile or peppermint, can soothe the digestive tract and alleviate discomfort.
- **Clear juices:** Opt for diluted fruit juices, such as apple or white grape juice, to provide energy and hydration.

- **Gelatin:** Low-sugar gelatin desserts can provide a source of protein and calories while remaining gentle on the digestive system.
- **Water:** Hydration is key during the acute phase, so be sure to drink plenty of water throughout the day.

What to Avoid:

- **Solid foods:** Avoid solid foods that may be difficult to digest and could exacerbate inflammation, such as raw fruits and vegetables, seeds, nuts, and tough meats.
- **Dairy products:** Dairy products, including milk, yogurt (but you can consider having plain Greek yogurt because they typically contain minimal fiber, around 0-1 gram per serving), and cheese, can be difficult for some individuals to tolerate during the acute phase and may worsen symptoms.
- **Caffeinated beverages:** Coffee, tea, and other caffeinated beverages can irritate the digestive tract and should be avoided.

Transitioning to Low-Fiber Food

As symptoms begin to improve and inflammation subsides, it's time to transition to a diet that includes low-fiber foods. These foods are easier to digest and less likely to cause irritation or discomfort in the digestive tract. Here are some tips for transitioning to low-fiber foods:

- **Start slowly:** Introduce low-fiber foods gradually to give your digestive system time to adjust. Begin with small portions and gradually increase the amount as tolerated.
- **Choose soft, cooked foods:** Opt for soft, cooked vegetables, such as carrots, squash, and potatoes, instead of raw or fibrous varieties.
- **Incorporate lean proteins:** Include lean proteins such as chicken, turkey, fish, and eggs in your diet to provide essential nutrients without added stress on the digestive system.
- **Avoid trigger foods:** Steer clear of foods that may trigger symptoms or exacerbate inflammation, such as spicy foods, fried foods, and high-fat dishes.

Tips for Managing Symptoms and Discomfort

Managing symptoms and discomfort during the acute phase of diverticulitis is essential for promoting healing and preventing complications. Here are some tips to help you cope with symptoms and improve your overall well-being:

- **Get plenty of rest:** Allow your body time to heal by getting adequate rest and avoiding strenuous activities.
- **Use heat therapy:** Applying a heating pad or warm compress to the abdomen can help alleviate abdominal pain and discomfort.
- **Stay hydrated:** Stay hydrated and aid in the healing process by consuming an ample amount of fluids, such as herbal teas, clear broths, and water.
- **Consider over-the-counter medications:** Over-the-counter pain relievers, such as acetaminophen or ibuprofen, may help alleviate discomfort. However, consult your healthcare provider before taking any medications to ensure they are safe for you.

Stage 2: Healing and Stabilization

Transitioning to Healing Foods

As you progress through your journey of managing diverticulitis, the healing and stabilization stage marks a significant milestone. During this phase, the focus shifts towards introducing healing foods that promote digestive health and support long-term well-being. Let's explore the essential strategies for transitioning to healing foods and building a balanced plate tailored to your needs.

Introduction of Low-Fiber Foods

During the healing and stabilization stage, the emphasis is on gradually reintroducing low-fiber foods into your diet. These foods are easier to digest and less likely to cause irritation or discomfort in the digestive tract. The following are some essential things to remember:

- **Start Slowly:** Begin by introducing small portions of low-fiber foods and gradually increase the amount as tolerated. This allows your digestive system time to adjust and minimizes the risk of symptoms flaring up.
- **Choose Cooked Vegetables:** Opt for soft, cooked vegetables such as carrots, squash, and potatoes instead of raw or fibrous varieties. Steaming or boiling vegetables can make them easier to digest.
- **Include Lean Proteins:** Incorporate lean proteins such as chicken, turkey, fish, eggs, and tofu into your meals to provide essential nutrients without added stress on the digestive system.
- **Incorporate Whole Grains:** Choose refined grains such as white rice, white bread, and pasta initially, and gradually reintroduce whole grains such as brown rice, whole wheat bread, and quinoa as tolerated.

Building a Balanced Plate

Creating a balanced plate is key to providing your body with the nutrients it needs to support healing and recovery. Aim to include a variety of foods from different food groups to ensure you're getting a well-rounded mix of nutrients. Here's how to build a balanced plate:

- **Fill Half Your Plate with Vegetables:** Vegetables are rich in vitamins, minerals, and antioxidants that support digestive health. Aim to fill half your plate with a variety of colorful vegetables, focusing on cooked or low-fiber options.
- **Add Lean Protein:** Include a serving of lean protein, such as grilled chicken, fish, tofu, or beans, to provide essential amino acids for tissue repair and muscle maintenance.
- **Incorporate Healthy Fats:** Include sources of healthy fats, such as avocado, nuts, seeds, and olive oil, to provide essential fatty acids and support overall health.
- **Include Whole Grains:** Incorporate a serving of whole grains, such as brown rice, quinoa, or whole wheat pasta, to provide fiber and sustained energy.

Foods to Emphasize and Foods to Limit

During the healing and stabilization stage, it's important to emphasize foods that support digestive health and limit those that may exacerbate symptoms or inflammation. Here are some foods to emphasize and limit:

Foods to Emphasize:

- **Fruits:** Soft, ripe fruits such as bananas, applesauce, and canned fruits without seeds or skins.
- **Vegetables:** Cooked or canned vegetables without seeds or skins, such as carrots, squash, and potatoes.
- **Lean Proteins:** Chicken, turkey, fish, eggs, tofu, and well-cooked beans and lentils.
- **Whole Grains:** Refined grains such as white rice, white bread, pasta, and crackers, and gradually reintroduce whole grains as tolerated.
- **Dairy:** Low-fat or non-fat dairy products such as milk, yogurt, and cheese.

Foods to Limit:

- **High-Fiber Foods:** Fibrous fruits and vegetables, whole grains, nuts, seeds, and legumes that may be difficult to digest.
- **Spicy Foods:** Spicy foods can irritate the digestive tract and exacerbate symptoms.
- **Fried and Greasy Foods:** High-fat foods can be hard to digest and may worsen symptoms such as bloating and abdominal discomfort.
- **Carbonated Beverages:** Carbonated beverages can cause gas and bloating, so it's best to limit or avoid them during this stage.

Stage 3: Maintenance and Prevention

Long-Term Dietary Strategies

Congratulations on reaching the maintenance and prevention stage of your diverticulitis management journey! This phase marks a crucial milestone in maintaining digestive health and preventing future flare-ups. Let's explore the key dietary strategies and lifestyle modifications tailored to support long-term well-being.

Gradual Introduction of High-Fiber Foods

During the maintenance and prevention stage, the focus shifts towards gradually reintroducing high-fiber foods into your diet. Fiber plays a crucial role in promoting regular bowel movements, preventing constipation, and reducing the risk of diverticulitis flare-ups. Here's how to incorporate high-fiber foods into your diet

- **Start Slowly:** Begin by introducing small portions of high-fiber foods and gradually increase the amount as tolerated. This allows your digestive system time to adjust and minimizes the risk of symptoms flaring up.
- **Choose Soluble Fiber:** Opt for soluble fiber sources such as fruits, vegetables, oats, and legumes, which are easier to digest and less likely to cause irritation in the digestive tract.
- **Include Insoluble Fiber:** Incorporate insoluble fiber sources such as whole grains, nuts, seeds, and bran gradually, as tolerated. These foods provide bulk to the stool and promote regular bowel movements.

Lifestyle Modifications for Prevention

In addition to dietary strategies, lifestyle modifications play a crucial role in preventing diverticulitis flare-ups and promoting overall well-being. Here are some key lifestyle modifications to consider:

- **Maintain a Healthy Weight:** Aim to maintain a healthy weight through a balanced diet and regular exercise. Excess weight can increase pressure within the colon and raise the risk of diverticulitis flare-ups.
- **Exercise Regularly:** Engage in regular physical activity, such as walking, jogging, swimming, or cycling, to promote digestive health and relieve stress.
- **Manage Stress:** Practice stress-reduction techniques such as deep breathing, meditation, yoga, or tai chi to reduce stress levels, which can trigger diverticulitis flare-ups.
- **Avoid Smoking:** If you smoke, consider quitting, as smoking is associated with an increased risk of diverticulitis and can exacerbate symptoms.

STAGE 1: ACUTE DIVERTICULITIS RECOVERY RECIPE

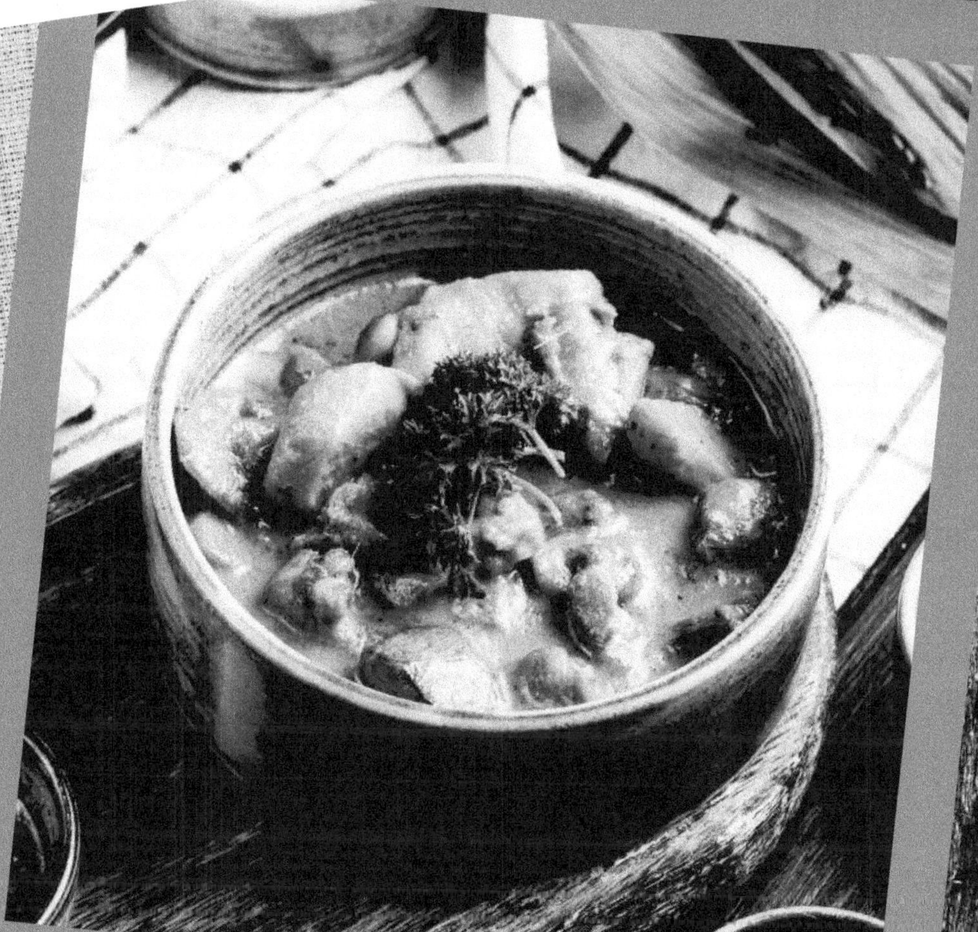

Breakfast Recipes

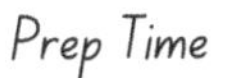
Prep Time

Cook Time

Rating

Difficulty

Instructions

Nutritional Value

Serving

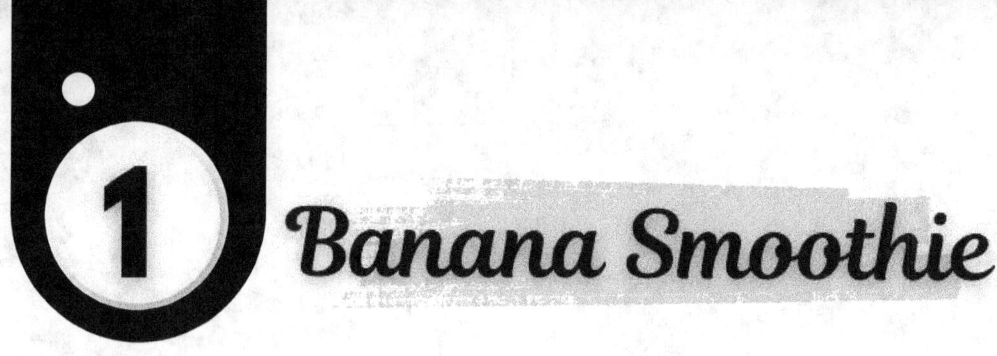

Banana Smoothie

Introduction

This creamy and soothing banana smoothie is a gentle and nourishing option for those in Stage 1 of diverticulitis recovery. Packed with potassium-rich bananas and easily digestible ingredients, it provides essential nutrients without irritating the digestive system.

Ingredients

- 2 ripe bananas
- 1 cup plain Greek yogurt
- 1/2 cup unsweetened almond milk (or any milk of your choice)
- 1 tablespoon honey (optional)
- Ice cubes (optional)

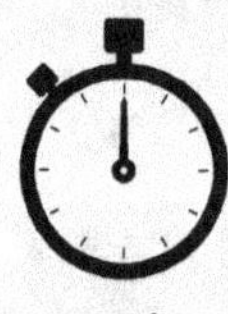

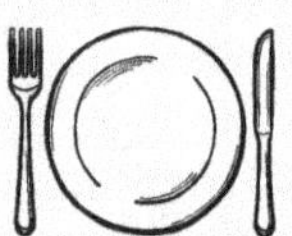

Prep Time	Cook Time	Serving
5 mins	0 mins	2

Preparation Method

1. Peel the bananas and cut them into chunks.

2. In a blender, combine the banana chunks, Greek yogurt, almond milk, and honey.

3. For a cooler consistency, feel free to add ice cubes.

4. Pour into glasses and serve immediately.

- Calories: 150 kcal
- Protein: 6g
- Fat: 2g
- Carbohydrates: 30g
- Fiber: 3g
- Sugar: 18g

Difficulty

Rating

Vegetable Broth

Introduction

A comforting and nourishing option during Stage 1 of diverticulitis recovery, vegetable broth provides hydration and essential nutrients without taxing the digestive system. This homemade version is free from artificial additives and can be customized with your favorite vegetables and herbs.

Ingredients

- 2 carrots, chopped
- 2 celery stalks, chopped
- 1 onion, chopped
- 2 cloves garlic, minced
- 6 cups water
- Salt and pepper to taste
- Fresh parsley or thyme (optional)

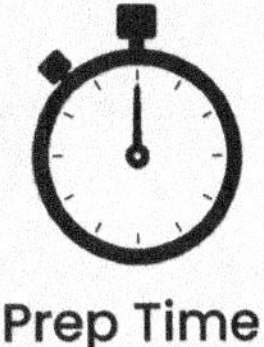
Prep Time
10 mins

Cook Time
45 mins

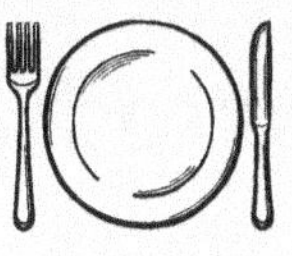
Serving
6 cups

Preparation Method

1. One tablespoon of olive oil should be heated over medium heat in a large pot.
2. Pour and add in the chopped carrots, celery, onion, and garlic to the pot. Sauté for 5-7 minutes until the vegetables are slightly softened.
3. Add the water and heat the mixture until it boils.
4. Reduce the heat to low and let the broth simmer for 30-45 minutes, uncovered.
5. Season with salt, pepper, and fresh herbs if desired.
6. Strain the broth through a fine-mesh sieve or cheesecloth to remove the solids.
7. Allow the broth to cool before storing it in airtight containers in the refrigerator or freezer.

- Calories: 15 kcal
- Protein: 0.5g
- Fat: 0g
- Carbohydrates: 3g
- Fiber: 1g
- Sugar: 1g

Difficulty

Rating

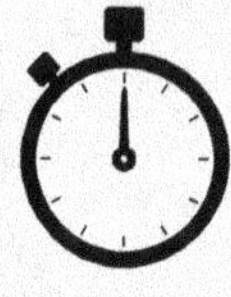
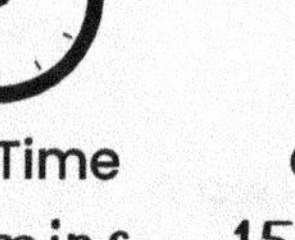

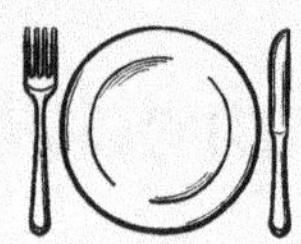

Applesauce

Introduction

Homemade applesauce is a gentle and soothing option for those in Stage 1 of diverticulitis recovery. Made with just a few simple ingredients, it provides comfort and hydration while being easy to digest.

Prep Time 10 mins

Cook Time 15-20 mins

Serving 2 cups

Ingredients

- 4 medium-sized apples (such as Gala or Fuji), peeled, cored, and chopped
- 1/2 cup water
- 1 tablespoon lemon juice
- 1-2 tablespoons honey or maple syrup (optional)
- 1/2 teaspoon ground cinnamon (optional)

Preparation Method

1. In a saucepan, combine the chopped apples, water, lemon juice, and optional sweetener and cinnamon.
2. After bringing the mixture to a boil over medium heat, lower the heat to a simmer and cover the pot. Simmer the apples for 15 to 20 minutes, or until they are tender and mashable.
3. Remove the saucepan from the heat and allow the applesauce to cool slightly.
4. Using a potato masher or fork, mash the cooked apples to your desired consistency. For a smoother texture, you can also blend the applesauce in a blender or food processor.
5. Taste and adjust the sweetness and seasoning if needed.
6. Transfer the applesauce to a jar or container and store it in the refrigerator for up to one week.

- Calories: 60 kcal
- Protein: 0g
- Fat: 0g
- Carbohydrates: 16g
- Fiber: 3g
- Sugar: 12g

Difficulty

Rating

Greek Yogurt With Honey

Introduction

Greek yogurt with honey is a creamy and protein-rich option for those in Stage 1 of diverticulitis recovery. With its smooth texture and natural sweetness, it provides essential nutrients while being gentle on the digestive system.

Ingredients

- 1 cup plain Greek yogurt
- 1-2 tablespoons honey (or to taste)
- Optional toppings: sliced bananas, berries, or chopped nuts

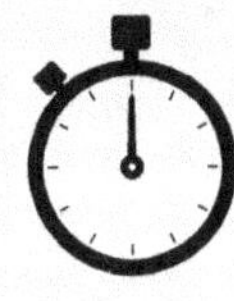

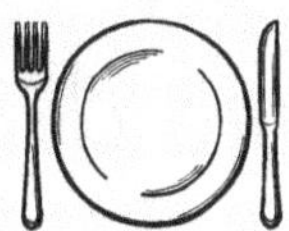

Prep Time
2 mins

Cook Time
0 mins

Serving
1

Preparation Method

1. Spoon Greek yogurt into a bowl.
2. Drizzle the honey over the yogurt, adjusting the amount to your desired sweetness.
3. Stir gently to combine.
4. If desired, top the yogurt with sliced bananas, berries, or chopped nuts for added flavor and texture.
5. Serve immediately and enjoy as a nourishing breakfast or snack.

- Calories: 150 kcal
- Protein: 18g
- Fat: 0g
- Carbohydrates: 20g
- Fiber: 0g
- Sugar: 18g

Difficulty

Rating

Rice Porridge

Introduction

Rice porridge, also known as congee, is a comforting and easily digestible option for individuals in Stage 1 of diverticulitis recovery. This simple dish is gentle on the digestive system while providing essential nutrients and hydration.

Ingredients

- 1/2 cup white rice (short or medium grain)
- 4 cups water or low-sodium chicken broth
- Salt to taste
- Optional toppings: sliced green onions, shredded chicken, soft-boiled egg, grated ginger

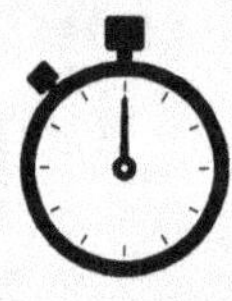 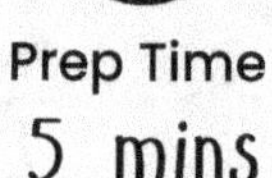  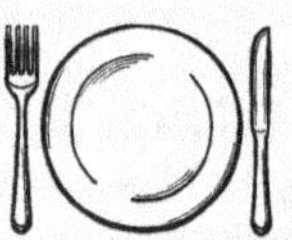

Prep Time	Cook Time	Serving
5 mins	30-40 mins	4

Preparation Method

1. Make sure the rice is thoroughly cleaned by running it under cold, and the water runs clear.
2. In a large pot, bring the water or chicken broth to a boil over medium-high heat.
3. Add the rinsed rice to the pot and stir to combine.
4. Reduce the heat to low and simmer, uncovered, stirring occasionally, for 30-40 minutes or until the rice is soft and porridge-like in consistency.
5. Season with salt to taste.
6. Serve the rice porridge hot, garnished with your choice of optional toppings, such as sliced green onions, shredded chicken, soft-boiled egg, or grated ginger.

- Calories: 150 kcal
- Protein: 3g
- Fat: 0g
- Carbohydrates: 33g
- Fiber: 0g
- Sugar: 0g

Difficulty

Rating

Scrambled Eggs

Introduction

Scrambled eggs are a gentle and protein-rich option for individuals in Stage 1 of diverticulitis recovery. This simple dish is easy to digest and can be customized with various ingredients to suit your preferences.

Ingredients

- 4 large eggs
- 2 tablespoons milk or water
- Salt and pepper to taste
- 1 tablespoon unsalted butter or olive oil
- Optional additions: diced vegetables (such as bell peppers, onions, or spinach), grated cheese, chopped herbs

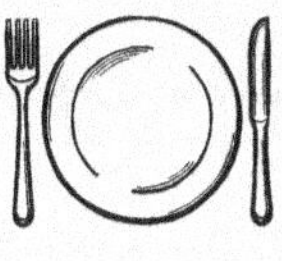

Prep Time 5 mins

Cook Time 5 mins

Serving 2

Preparation Method

1. In a bowl, whisk together the eggs, milk or water, salt, and pepper until well combined.
2. Heat the butter or olive oil in a non-stick skillet over medium heat.
3. Pour the egg mixture into the skillet and let it cook undisturbed for a few seconds until the edges start to set.
4. Using a spatula, gently push the cooked edges toward the center of the skillet, allowing the uncooked eggs to flow to the edges.
5. Continue to cook and gently stir the eggs until they are just set and slightly creamy in texture.
6. Remove the skillet from the heat and transfer the scrambled eggs to a plate.
7. Serve immediately, garnished with your choice of optional additions, such as diced vegetables, grated cheese, or chopped herbs

- Calories: 160 kcal
- Protein: 10g
- Fat: 12g
- Carbohydrates: 2g
- Fiber: 0g
- Sugar: 1g

Difficulty

Rating

Oatmeal Porridge

Introduction

Oatmeal porridge is a comforting and nourishing option for individuals in Stage 1 of diverticulitis recovery. This gentle dish is easy to digest and provides essential nutrients to support healing and recovery.

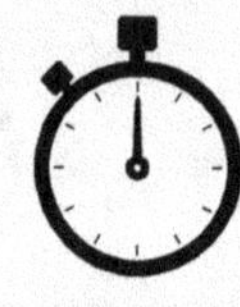
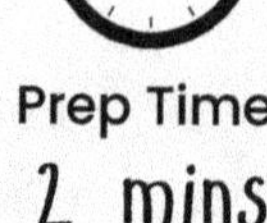

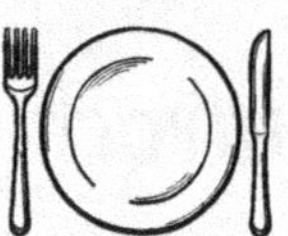

Prep Time	Cook Time	Serving
2 mins	5-7 mins	1

Preparation Method

1. In a small saucepan, bring the water or milk to a boil over medium-high heat.
2. Stir in the oats and salt, then reduce the heat to low.
3. Simmer the oats, stirring occasionally, for 5-7 minutes or until thick and creamy.
4. Remove the saucepan from the heat and let the oatmeal rest for a minute or two.
5. Serve the oatmeal hot, topped with your choice of optional toppings, such as sliced banana, berries, chopped nuts, or a drizzle of honey or maple syrup.

Ingredients

- 1/2 cup old-fashioned oats
- 1 cup water or milk (dairy or plant-based)
- Pinch of salt
- Optional toppings: sliced banana, berries, chopped nuts, honey or maple syrup

- Calories: 150 kcal
- Protein: 5g
- Fat: 3g
- Carbohydrates: 27g
- Fiber: 4g
- Sugar: 1g

Difficulty

Rating

Cream of Wheat

Introduction

Cream of Wheat is a comforting and easily digestible option for individuals in Stage 1 of diverticulitis recovery. This warm cereal provides essential nutrients and can be customized with various toppings to suit your preferences.

Ingredients

- 1/4 cup Cream of Wheat cereal
- 1 cup water or milk (dairy or plant-based)
- Pinch of salt
- Optional toppings: sliced banana, berries, honey or maple syrup

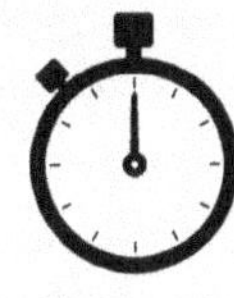

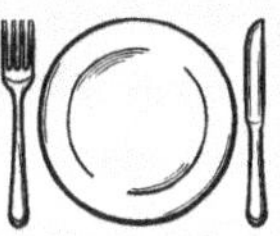

Prep Time
1 mins

Cook Time
2-3 mins

Serving
1

Preparation Method

1. In a small saucepan, bring the water or milk to a boil over medium-high heat.
2. Slowly add the Cream of Wheat cereal to the boiling liquid, stirring constantly to prevent lumps from forming.
3. Reduce the heat to low and simmer the cereal, stirring occasionally, for 2-3 minutes or until thickened to your desired consistency.
4. Remove the saucepan from the heat and let the Cream of Wheat cool slightly.
5. Serve the Cream of Wheat hot, topped with your choice of optional toppings, such as sliced banana, berries, chopped nuts, or a drizzle of honey or maple syrup.

- Calories: 100 kcal
- Protein: 3g
- Fat: 0g
- Carbohydrates: 22g
- Fiber: 1g
- Sugar: 0g

Difficulty

Rating

STAGE 1: ACUTE DIVERTICULITIS RECOVERY RECIPE

Lunch Recipes

Prep Time | Cook Time | Rating | Difficulty | Instructions | Nutritional Value | Serving

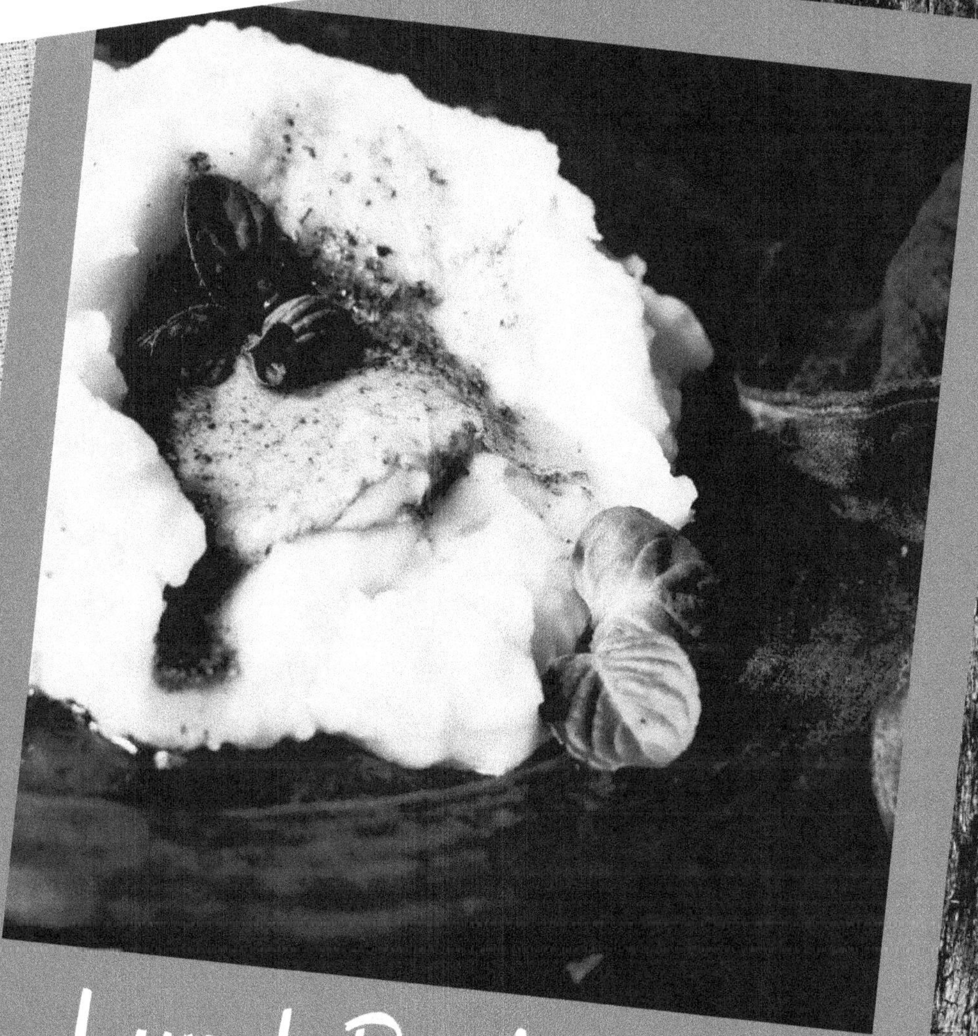

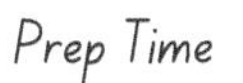

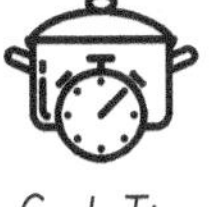

Clear Chicken Broth

Introduction

Clear chicken broth is a soothing and nourishing option for individuals in Stage 1 of diverticulitis recovery. This gentle broth provides hydration and essential nutrients without taxing the digestive system.

Ingredients

- 2 boneless, skinless chicken breasts
- 8 cups water
- 1 onion, peeled and quartered
- 2 carrots, peeled and chopped
- 2 celery stalks, chopped
- 2 cloves garlic, smashed
- 1 bay leaf
- Salt to taste
- Fresh parsley for garnish (optional)

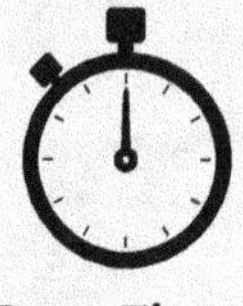

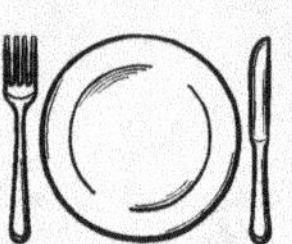

Prep Time 10 mins **Cook Time** 1-1.5 hours **Serving** 8 cups

Preparation Method

1. In a large pot, combine the chicken breasts, water, onion, carrots, celery, garlic, and bay leaf.
2. Bring the mixture to a boil over medium-high heat, then reduce the heat to low and simmer, uncovered, for 1-1.5 hours, skimming off any foam that rises to the surface.
3. Remove the chicken breasts from the pot and set them aside to cool slightly.
4. Strain the broth through a fine-mesh sieve or cheesecloth into a clean pot.
5. Season the broth with salt to taste.
6. Once the chicken breasts have cooled, shred the meat using two forks and add it back to the broth.
7. Reheat the broth over low heat until warmed through.
8. Serve the clear chicken broth hot, garnished with fresh parsley if desired.

- Calories: 50 kcal
- Protein: 6g
- Fat: 1g
- Carbohydrates: 3g
- Fiber: 1g
- Sugar: 1g

Difficulty

Rating

Herbal Tea With Lemon

Introduction

Herbal tea with lemon is a comforting and hydrating option for individuals in Stage 1 of diverticulitis recovery. This soothing beverage provides warmth and essential nutrients without irritating the digestive system.

Ingredients

- 1 herbal tea bag (such as chamomile, peppermint, or ginger)
- 1 cup boiling water
- Fresh lemon slices (optional)
- Honey or stevia (optional)

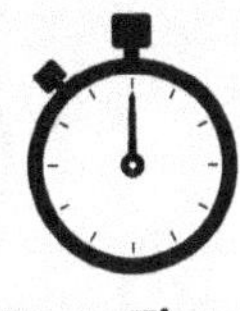

Prep Time
1 mins

Cook Time
5-7 mins

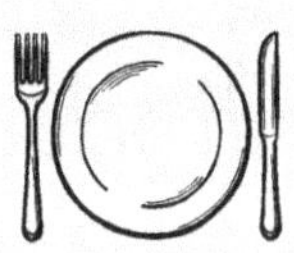

Serving
1

Preparation Method

1. Place the herbal tea bag in a heatproof mug.
2. Over the tea bag, pour the boiling water.
3. Let the tea steep for 5-7 minutes or according to package instructions.
4. Remove the tea bag and discard.
5. If desired, add fresh lemon slices and honey or stevia to taste.
6. Stir well and serve the herbal tea hot.

- Calories: 0 kcal
- Protein: 0g
- Fat: 0g
- Carbohydrates: 0g
- Fiber: 0g
- Sugar: 0g

Difficulty

Rating

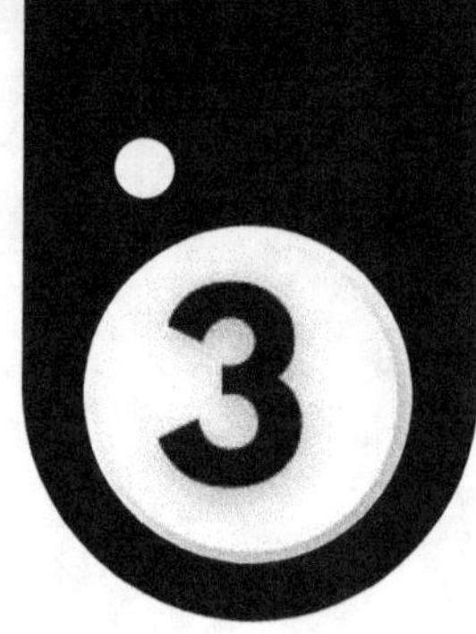

Clear Vegetable Broth With Steamed Carrots

Introduction

Clear vegetable broth with steamed carrots is a gentle and nourishing option for individuals in Stage 1 of diverticulitis recovery. This soothing broth provides hydration and essential nutrients, while the steamed carrots add a touch of flavor and texture.

Ingredients

- 4 cups water
- 1 onion, peeled and quartered
- 2 carrots, peeled and chopped
- 2 celery stalks, chopped
- 2 cloves garlic, smashed
- 1 bay leaf
- Salt to taste
- Fresh parsley for garnish (optional)

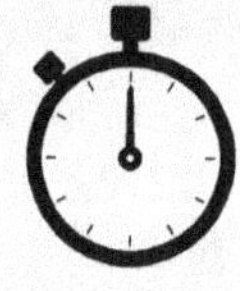 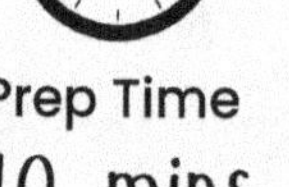  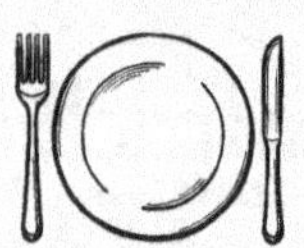

Prep Time
10 mins

Cook Time
45-60 mins

Serving
4

Preparation Method

1. In a large pot, combine the water, onion, carrots, celery, garlic, and bay leaf.
2. Bring the mixture to a boil over medium-high heat, then reduce the heat to low and simmer, uncovered, for 45-60 minutes.
3. Strain the broth through a fine-mesh sieve or cheesecloth into a clean pot.
4. Season the broth with salt to taste.
5. Meanwhile, steam the chopped carrots until tender, about 5-7 minutes.
6. Divide the steamed carrots among serving bowls.
7. Ladle the clear vegetable broth over the steamed carrots.
8. Garnish with fresh parsley, if desired.
9. Serve the clear vegetable broth with steamed carrots hot.

- Calories: 15 kcal
- Protein: 0g
- Fat: 0g
- Carbohydrates: 3g
- Fiber: 1g
- Sugar: 1g

Difficulty

Rating

Fruit Gelatin Cups

Introduction

Fruit gelatin cups are a light and refreshing option for individuals in Stage 1 of diverticulitis recovery. Made with clear gelatin and fruit juice, these colorful cups provide hydration and a hint of sweetness without irritating the digestive system.

Ingredients

- 2 cups clear fruit juice (such as apple, white grape, or pear)
- 2 packets unflavored gelatin
- Fresh fruit slices for garnish (optional)

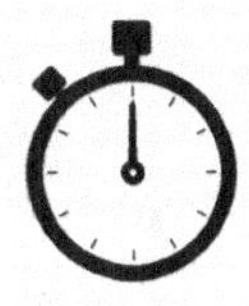
Prep Time
5 mins

Cook Time
5 mins
+
Chilling time

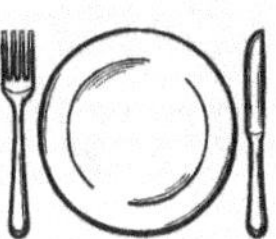
Serving
4

Preparation Method

1. In a small saucepan, heat 1 cup of the fruit juice over low heat until warm but not boiling.
2. Sprinkle the unflavored gelatin over the warm fruit juice and stir until completely dissolved.
3. Remove the saucepan from the heat and stir in the remaining 1 cup of fruit juice.
4. Divide the mixture among serving cups or molds.
5. Refrigerate the gelatin cups for 4-6 hours or until set.
6. Once set, garnish the gelatin cups with fresh fruit slices, if desired.
7. Serve the fruit gelatin cups chilled.

- Calories: 60 kcal
- Protein: 2g
- Fat: 0g
- Carbohydrates: 14g
- Fiber: 0g
- Sugar: 14g

Difficulty

Rating

Apple Juice

Introduction

Apple juice is a gentle and hydrating option for individuals in Stage 1 of diverticulitis recovery. This refreshing beverage provides essential nutrients and can be enjoyed on its own or mixed with water for a lighter flavor.

Ingredients

- 2-3 apples, cored and chopped
- Water

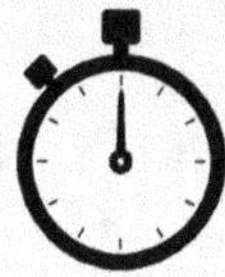

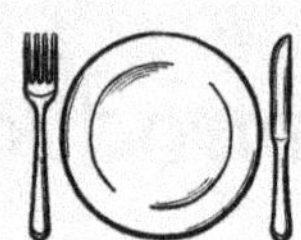

Prep Time
5 mins

Cook Time
0 mins

Serving
2 cups

Preparation Method

1. Place the chopped apples in a blender or food processor.
2. Add a small amount of water to help with blending, about 1/4 cup.
3. Blend the apples until smooth.
4. Strain the blended apples through a fine-mesh sieve or cheesecloth to remove the pulp.
5. Discard the pulp and transfer the strained apple juice to a clean container.
6. Serve the apple juice chilled or over ice, if desired.

- Calories: 120 kcal
- Protein: 0g
- Fat: 0g
- Carbohydrates: 30g
- Fiber: 3g
- Sugar: 25g

Difficulty

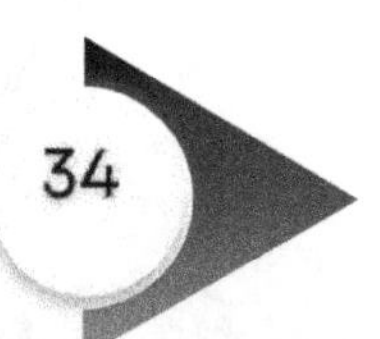

Rating

Green Tea
With Honey

Introduction

Green tea with honey is a soothing and antioxidant-rich option for individuals in Stage 1 of diverticulitis recovery. This warm beverage provides hydration and a touch of sweetness without irritating the digestive system.

Prep Time
1 mins

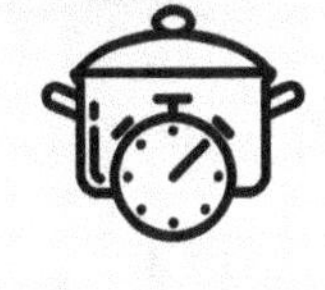

Cook Time
3-5 mins
(steeping time)

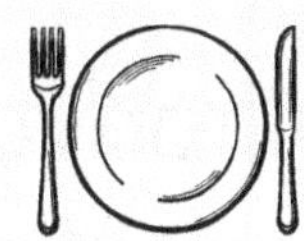

Serving
1

Ingredients

- 1 green tea bag
- 1 cup boiling water
- 1 teaspoon honey (or to taste)

Preparation Method

1. Place the green tea bag in a heatproof mug.
2. Over the tea bag, pour the boiling water.
3. Let the tea steep for 3-5 minutes or according to package instructions.
4. Remove the tea bag and discard.
5. Stir in the honey until dissolved.
6. Serve the green tea with honey hot.

- Calories: 20 kcal
- Protein: 0g
- Fat: 0g
- Carbohydrates: 5g
- Fiber: 0g
- Sugar: 5g

Difficulty

Rating

Citrus Gelatin Mold

Introduction

Citrus gelatin mold is a light and refreshing option for individuals in Stage 1 of diverticulitis recovery. This gentle dessert provides hydration and a burst of citrus flavor without irritating the digestive system.

Ingredients

- 2 cups citrus juice (such as orange, grapefruit, or a combination)
- 2 packets unflavored gelatin
- 1 tablespoon honey or maple syrup (optional)
- Fresh citrus slices for garnish (optional)

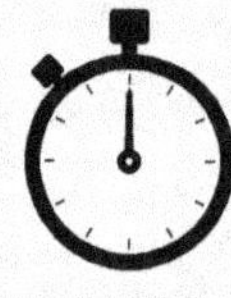 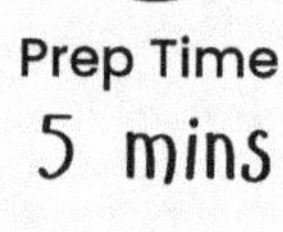
Prep Time
5 mins

Cook Time
5 mins
+
(steeping time)

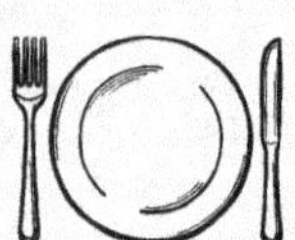
Serving
4

Preparation Method

1. In a small saucepan, heat 1 cup of the citrus juice over low heat until warm but not boiling.
2. Sprinkle the unflavored gelatin over the warm citrus juice and stir until completely dissolved.
3. Remove the saucepan from the heat and stir in the remaining 1 cup of citrus juice.
4. If desired, sweeten the mixture with honey or maple syrup to taste.
5. Pour the mixture into a gelatin mold or individual serving cups.
6. Refrigerate the gelatin mold for 4-6 hours or until set.
7. Once set, garnish with fresh citrus slices, if desired.
8. Serve the citrus gelatin mold chilled.

- Calories: 60 kcal
- Protein: 2g
- Fat: 0g
- Carbohydrates: 14g
- Fiber: 0g
- Sugar: 12g

Difficulty

Rating

Mashed Butternut Squash

Introduction

Mashed butternut squash is a comforting and nourishing option for individuals in Stage 1 of diverticulitis recovery. This soft and creamy dish provides essential nutrients and is easy to digest.

Ingredients

- 1 medium butternut squash, peeled, seeded, and diced
- Water
- Salt to taste
- Butter or olive oil for serving (optional)

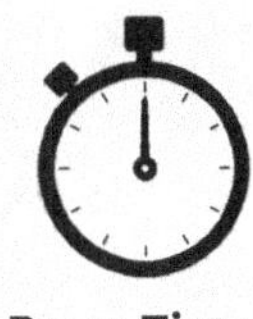  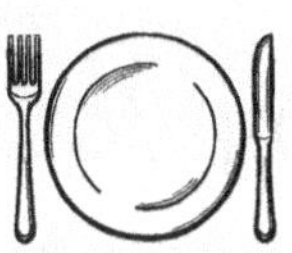

Prep Time 10 mins **Cook Time** 15-20 mins **Serving** Approx. 4

Preparation Method

1. Place the diced butternut squash in a large pot and cover with water.
2. Bring the water to a boil over medium-high heat, then reduce the heat to low and simmer for 15-20 minutes or until the squash is tender.
3. Drain the cooked squash and transfer it to a mixing bowl.
4. Use a potato masher or fork to mash the squash until smooth and creamy.
5. Season the mashed squash with salt to taste.
6. Serve the mashed butternut squash hot, with a pat of butter or drizzle of olive oil, if desired.

- Calories: 80 kcal
- Protein: 2g
- Fat: 0g
- Carbohydrates: 20g
- Fiber: 4g
- Sugar: 4g

Difficulty

Rating

Steamed White Fish

Introduction

Steamed white fish is a gentle and easily digestible option for individuals in Stage 1 of diverticulitis recovery. This delicate dish provides lean protein and essential nutrients without putting stress on the digestive system.

Ingredients

- 4 white fish fillets (such as tilapia, cod, or sole)
- Salt and pepper to taste
- Lemon wedges for serving (optional)
- Fresh herbs for garnish (optional)

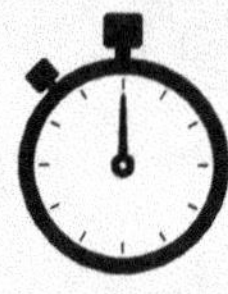

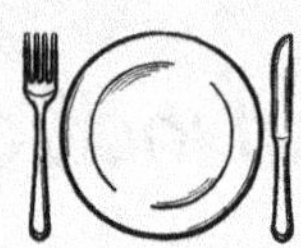

Prep Time
5 mins

Cook Time
8-10 mins

Serving
4

Preparation Method

1. Season the white fish fillets with salt and pepper to taste.
2. Place the seasoned fish fillets in a single layer in a steamer basket or on a plate that fits inside a steamer.
3. Fill a pot with water and bring it to a simmer over medium-high heat.
4. Place the steamer basket or plate with the fish over the simmering water, ensuring that the water does not touch the fish.
5. Cover the pot with a lid and steam the fish for 8-10 minutes or until opaque and cooked through.
6. Carefully remove the steamed fish from the steamer and transfer to serving plates.
7. Serve the steamed white fish hot, with lemon wedges and fresh herbs for garnish, if desired.

- Calories: 120 kcal
- Protein: 25g
- Fat: 2g
- Carbohydrates: 0g
- Fiber: 0g
- Sugar: 0g

Difficulty

Rating

Boiled Egg
With Steamed Spinach

Introduction

Boiled eggs with steamed spinach are a gentle and nourishing option for individuals in Stage 1 of diverticulitis recovery. This protein-rich dish provides essential nutrients and fiber from the spinach, all while being easy on the digestive system.

Ingredients

- 4 eggs
- 2 cups fresh spinach leaves, washed
- Salt and pepper to taste

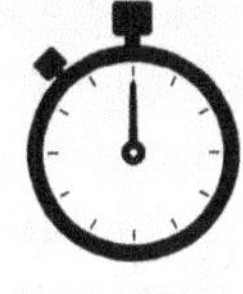

Prep Time

5 mins

Cook Time

8-10 mins(eegs)

2-3 mins(spinach)

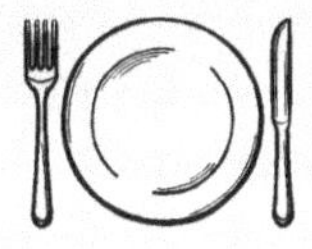

Serving

2

Preparation Method

1. Put the eggs in a saucepan and pour cold water over them.
2. Heat the water on medium-high until it boils.
3. Once boiling, reduce the heat to low and simmer the eggs for 8-10 minutes for hard-boiled eggs or 4-5 minutes for soft-boiled eggs.
4. While the eggs are cooking, prepare a steamer basket over a pot of boiling water.
5. Place the fresh spinach leaves in the steamer basket and steam for 2-3 minutes or until wilted.
6. Remove the spinach from the steamer and season with salt and pepper to taste.
7. Once the eggs are cooked to your desired doneness, remove them from the saucepan and transfer them to a bowl of cold water to cool.
8. Peel the eggs and slice them in half.
9. Serve the boiled eggs with steamed spinach alongside.

- Calories: 160 kcal
- Protein: 12g
- Fat: 11g
- Carbohydrates: 3g
- Fiber: 2g
- Sugar: 0g

Difficulty

Rating

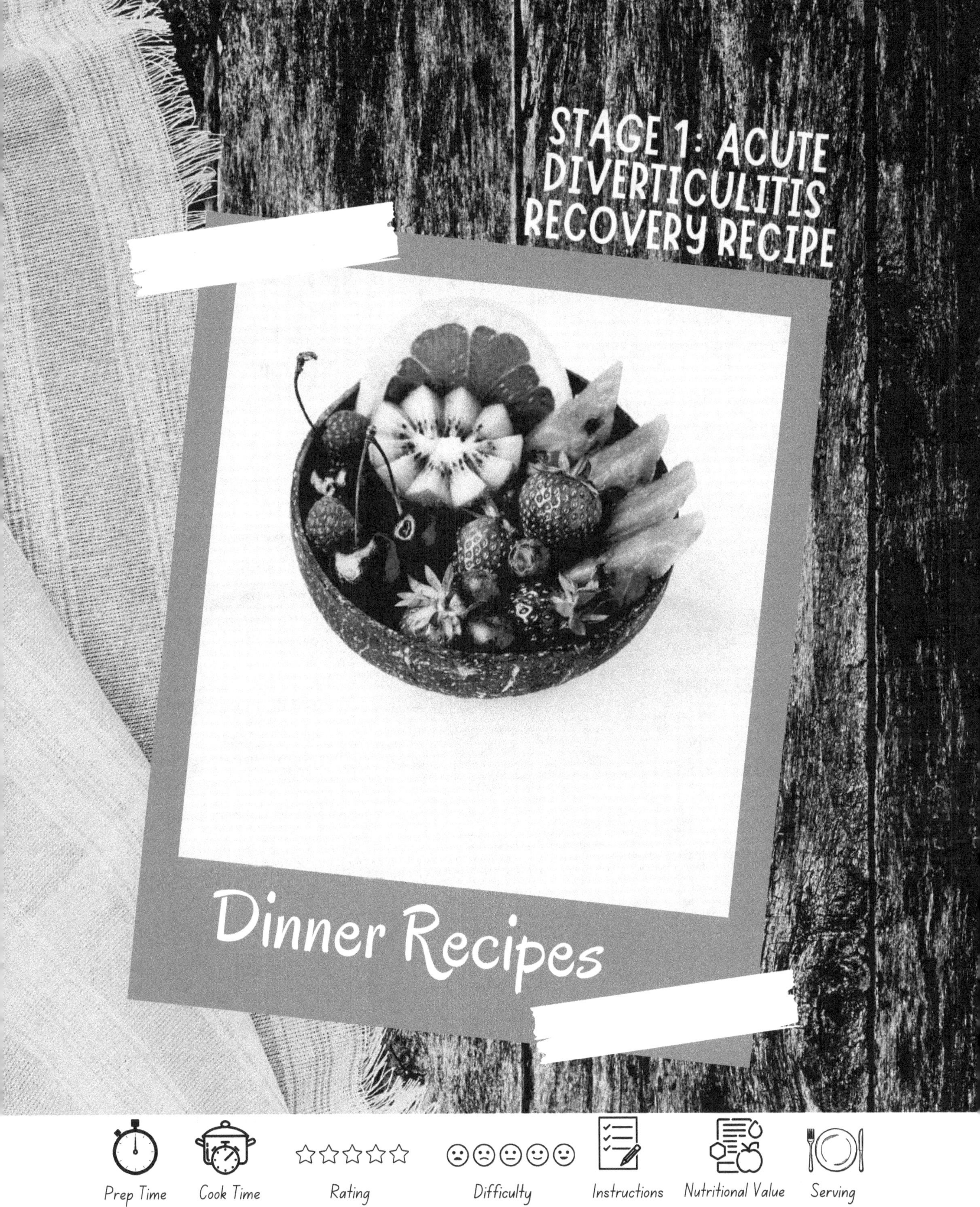

Dinner Recipes

Prep Time   Cook Time   Rating   Difficulty   Instructions   Nutritional Value   Serving

Clear Vegetable Broth *With* Steamed Green Beans

Introduction

Clear vegetable broth with steamed green beans is a gentle and nourishing option for individuals in Stage 1 of diverticulitis recovery. This soothing broth provides hydration and essential nutrients, while the steamed green beans add a touch of flavor and texture without irritating the digestive system.

Ingredients

- 4 cups water
- 1 onion, peeled and quartered
- 2 carrots, peeled and chopped
- 2 celery stalks, chopped
- 2 cloves garlic, smashed
- 1 bay leaf
- Salt to taste
- 1 cup fresh green beans, trimmed

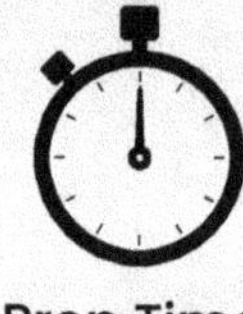  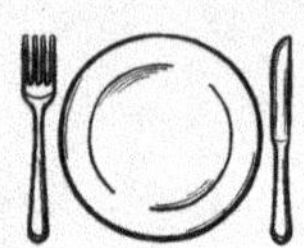

Prep Time
10 mins

Cook Time
45-60 mins

Serving
4

Preparation Method

1. In a large pot, combine the water, onion, carrots, celery, garlic, and bay leaf.
2. Bring the mixture to a boil over medium-high heat, then reduce the heat to low and simmer, uncovered, for 45-60 minutes.
3. Strain the broth through a fine-mesh sieve or cheesecloth into a clean pot.
4. Season the broth with salt to taste.
5. Meanwhile, steam the green beans until tender, about 5-7 minutes.
6. Divide the steamed green beans among serving bowls.
7. Ladle the clear vegetable broth over the steamed green beans.
8. Serve the clear vegetable broth with steamed green beans hot.

- Calories: 15 kcal
- Protein: 1g
- Fat: 0g
- Carbohydrates: 3g
- Fiber: 1g
- Sugar: 1g

Difficulty

Rating

Herbal Infusion With Soft Tofu

Introduction

Herbal infusion with soft tofu is a comforting and nourishing option for individuals in Stage 1 of diverticulitis recovery. This warm beverage provides hydration and a boost of protein from the tofu, while the herbal infusion adds soothing properties to help ease digestive discomfort.

Ingredients

- 2 cups water
- 1 herbal tea bag (such as chamomile or peppermint)
- 1/2 cup soft tofu, cubed
- Honey or maple syrup to taste (optional)

  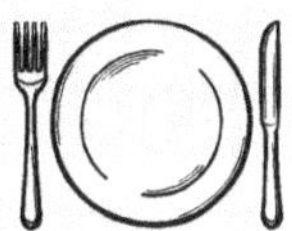

Prep Time
5 mins

Cook Time
5 mins
(Plus steeping time)

Serving
2

Preparation Method

1. In a small saucepan, bring the water to a boil over medium-high heat.
2. Remove the saucepan from the heat and add the herbal tea bag.
3. Let the tea steep for 3-5 minutes or according to package instructions.
4. Remove the tea bag and discard.
5. Divide the cubed soft tofu among serving cups.
6. Pour the herbal infusion over the tofu.
7. If desired, sweeten the herbal infusion with honey or maple syrup to taste.
8. Serve the herbal infusion with soft tofu warm

- Calories: 30 kcal
- Protein: 2g
- Fat: 1g
- Carbohydrates: 2g
- Fiber: 0g
- Sugar: 1g

Difficulty

Rating

Mashed Pumpkin With Rice

Introduction

Mashed pumpkin with rice is a comforting and nourishing option for individuals in Stage 1 of diverticulitis recovery. This soft and creamy dish provides essential nutrients and gentle fiber from the pumpkin and rice, all while being easy on the digestive system.

Ingredients

- 1 small pumpkin, peeled, seeded, and cubed
- 1 cup white rice
- Water
- Salt to taste
- Butter or olive oil for serving (optional)

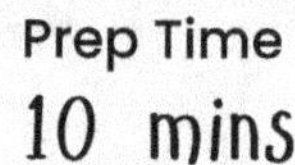

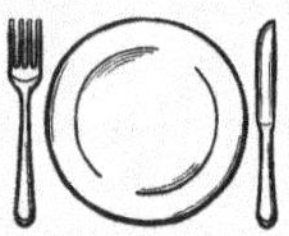

Prep Time
10 mins

Cook Time
30-40 mins

Serving
4

Preparation Method

1. Place the cubed pumpkin in a large pot and cover with water.
2. Bring the water to a boil over medium-high heat, then reduce the heat to low and simmer for 15-20 minutes or until the pumpkin is tender.
3. While the pumpkin is cooking, rinse the rice under cold water until the water runs clear.
4. In a separate pot, combine the rinsed rice with 2 cups of water and a pinch of salt.
5. Bring the rice to a boil, then reduce the heat to low and simmer, covered, for 15-20 minutes or until the rice is cooked and fluffy.
6. Drain the cooked pumpkin and transfer it to a mixing bowl.
7. Use a potato masher or fork to mash the pumpkin until smooth and creamy.
8. Serve the mashed pumpkin with cooked rice, seasoned with salt to taste.
9. Optionally, add a pat of butter or drizzle of olive oil for extra flavor.

- Calories: 200 kcal
- Protein: 4g
- Fat: 1g
- Carbohydrates: 45g
- Fiber: 4g
- Sugar: 4g

Difficulty

Rating

4 — Clear Beef Consommé With Soft Noodles

Introduction

Clear beef consommé with soft noodles is a comforting and nourishing option for individuals in Stage 1 of diverticulitis recovery. This flavorful broth provides hydration and essential nutrients, while the soft noodles add texture without irritating the digestive system.

Ingredients

- 4 cups beef broth
- 1 cup soft noodles (such as egg noodles or rice noodles)
- Salt and pepper to taste
- Fresh parsley for garnish (optional)

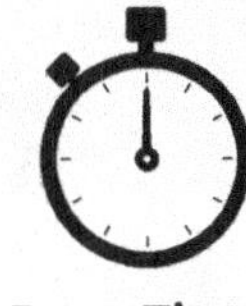
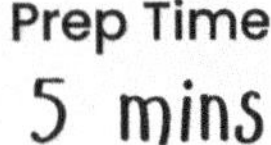

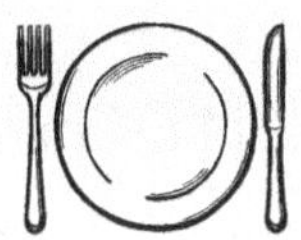

Prep Time
5 mins

Cook Time
10-15 mins

Serving
Approx. 4

Preparation Method

1. In a large pot, bring the beef broth to a boil over medium-high heat.
2. Add the soft noodles to the boiling broth and cook according to package instructions until tender.
3. Season the broth with salt and pepper to taste.
4. Once the noodles are cooked, remove the pot from the heat.
5. Ladle the clear beef consommé with soft noodles into serving bowls.
6. Garnish with fresh parsley, if desired.
7. Serve the clear beef consommé with soft noodles hot.

- Calories: 150 kcal
- Protein: 6g
- Fat: 1g
- Carbohydrates: 30g
- Fiber: 2g
- Sugar: 1g

Difficulty

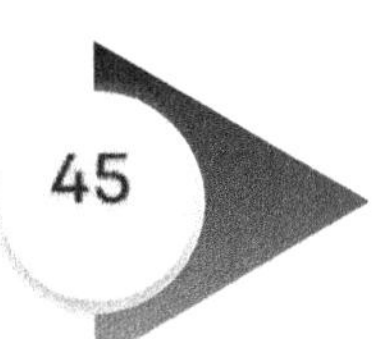

Rating

5 Jellied Cranberry Sauce With Greek Yogurt

Introduction

Jellied cranberry sauce with Greek yogurt is a delightful and soothing option for individuals in Stage 1 of diverticulitis recovery. This combination provides a balance of sweet and tangy flavors, along with the probiotic benefits of Greek yogurt, making it gentle on the digestive system.

Ingredients

- 1 cup jellied cranberry sauce
- 1/2 cup Greek yogurt
- Fresh mint leaves for garnish (optional)

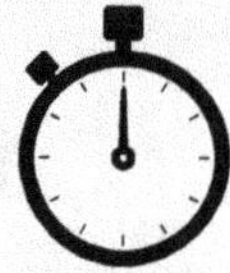

Prep Time
5 mins

Cook Time
0 mins

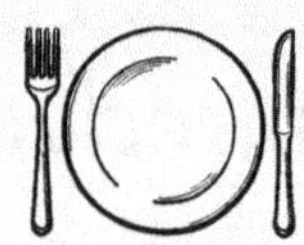

Serving
2

Preparation Method

1. Spoon the jellied cranberry sauce into serving bowls.

2. Add a dollop of Greek yogurt on top of the cranberry sauce in each bowl.

3. If preferred, garnish with fresh mint leaves.

4. Serve the jellied cranberry sauce with Greek yogurt chilled.

- Calories: 100 kcal
- Protein: 3g
- Fat: 0g
- Carbohydrates: 20g
- Fiber: 1g
- Sugar: 15g

Difficulty

Rating

6 Apple Cider with Boiled Potatoes

Introduction

Apple cider with boiled potatoes is a comforting and nourishing option for individuals in Stage 1 of diverticulitis recovery. This combination provides hydration and essential nutrients, along with the gentle texture of boiled potatoes, making it easy on the digestive system.

Ingredients

- 2 cups apple cider
- 2 medium potatoes, peeled and diced
- Salt to taste
- Fresh parsley for garnish (optional)

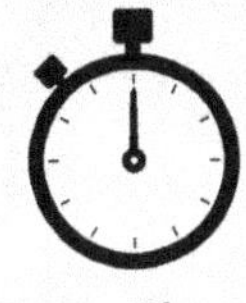

Prep Time
5 mins

Cook Time
15-20 mins

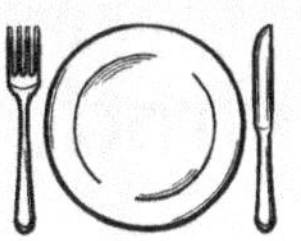

Serving
2

Preparation Method

1. In a small saucepan, bring the apple cider to a simmer over medium heat.
2. Meanwhile, place the diced potatoes in a separate pot and cover with water.
3. Bring the water to a boil over medium-high heat, then reduce the heat to low and simmer the potatoes for 10-15 minutes or until tender.
4. Drain the cooked potatoes and transfer them to serving bowls.
5. Once the apple cider is warmed through, pour it over the boiled potatoes in the serving bowls.
6. Season with salt to taste.
7. Garnish with fresh parsley, if desired.
8. Serve the apple cider with boiled potatoes warm.

- Calories: 150 kcal
- Protein: 2g
- Fat: 0g
- Carbohydrates: 35g
- Fiber: 3g
- Sugar: 20g

Difficulty

Rating

Lemon Infused Water With Scrambled Eggs

Introduction

Lemon-infused water with scrambled eggs is a refreshing and nourishing option for individuals in Stage 1 of diverticulitis recovery. This combination provides hydration and protein, along with a touch of citrus flavor from the lemon, making it gentle on the digestive system.

Ingredients

- 2 cups water
- 1 lemon, sliced
- 4 eggs
- Salt and pepper to taste
- Fresh chives for garnish (optional)

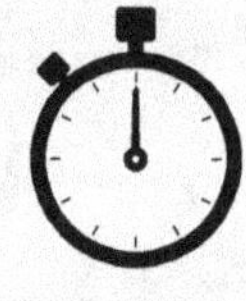

Prep Time
5 mins
(plus chilling time for the infused water)

Cook Time
5 mins

Serving
2

Preparation Method

1. In a pitcher, combine the water with the sliced lemon.

2. Let the lemon-infused water sit in the refrigerator for at least 1 hour to allow the flavors to meld.

3. When ready to serve, crack the eggs into a bowl and whisk until well beaten.

4. Heat a non-stick skillet over medium heat and pour in the beaten eggs.

5. Stir the eggs gently with a spatula, cooking until they are scrambled and cooked through.

6. Season the scrambled eggs with salt and pepper to taste.

7. Divide the scrambled eggs among serving plates.

8. Pour the lemon-infused water into glasses and serve alongside the scrambled eggs.

9. Garnish the scrambled eggs with fresh chives, if desired.

- Calories: 180 kcal
- Protein: 12g
- Fat: 12g
- Carbohydrates: 4g
- Fiber: 1g
- Sugar: 1g

Difficulty

Rating

Soft Polenta With Cooked Carrots

Introduction

Soft polenta with cooked carrots is a comforting and nourishing option for individuals in Stage 1 of diverticulitis recovery. This creamy dish provides hydration and gentle fiber from the polenta and carrots, making it easy on the digestive system.

Ingredients

- 1/2 cup polenta (cornmeal)
- 2 cups water
- Pinch of salt
- 2 carrots, peeled and diced
- Butter or olive oil for serving (optional)

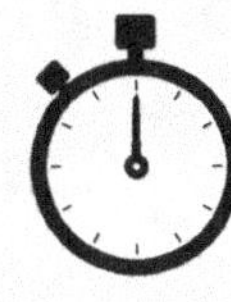
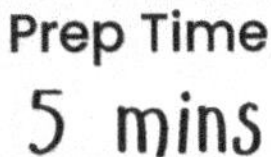

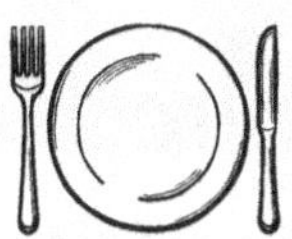

Prep Time
5 mins

Cook Time
25-30 mins

Serving
2

Preparation Method

1. In a saucepan, bring the water to a boil over medium-high heat.
2. To avoid lumps, gradually whisk in the polenta while stirring continually.
3. Reduce the heat to low and simmer, stirring occasionally, for 15-20 minutes or until the polenta is thick and creamy.
4. Meanwhile, place the diced carrots in a separate pot and cover with water.
5. Bring the water to a boil over medium-high heat, then reduce the heat to low and simmer the carrots for 10-15 minutes or until tender.
6. Drain the cooked carrots and set aside.
7. Once the polenta is cooked, season it with a pinch of salt and stir in the cooked carrots.
8. Divide the soft polenta with cooked carrots among serving bowls.
9. Optionally, top with a pat of butter or drizzle of olive oil for extra flavor.

- Calories: 150 kcal
- Protein: 3g
- Fat: 1g
- Carbohydrates: 30g
- Fiber: 4g
- Sugar: 2g

Difficulty

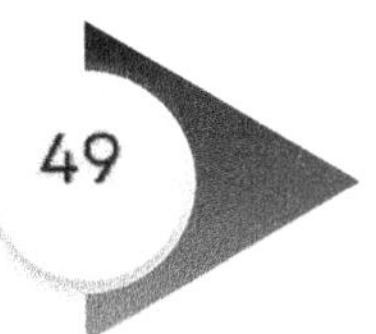

Rating

9

Pear Juice
With Baked Chicken Breast

Introduction

Pear juice with baked chicken breast is a nourishing and satisfying option for individuals in Stage 1 of diverticulitis recovery. This combination provides hydration and protein, along with the gentle sweetness of pear juice, making it easy on the digestive system.

Ingredients

- 2 boneless, skinless chicken breasts
- Salt and pepper to taste
- 1 tablespoon olive oil
- 1 cup pear juice
- Fresh parsley for garnish (optional)

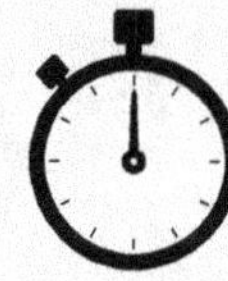  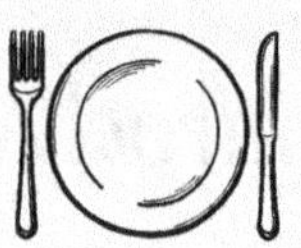

Prep Time
5 mins

Cook Time
25-30 mins

Serving
2

Preparation Method

1. Preheat the oven to 375°F (190°C).
2. Apply salt and pepper to both sides of the chicken breasts for seasoning.
3. Heat the olive oil in an oven-safe skillet over medium-high heat.
4. Add the seasoned chicken breasts to the skillet and sear for 2-3 minutes on each side until golden brown.
5. Transfer the skillet to the preheated oven and bake for 20-25 minutes or until the chicken is cooked through and reaches an internal temperature of 165°F (74°C).
6. Remove the chicken breasts from the oven and let them rest for a few minutes before slicing.
7. Divide the sliced chicken breasts among serving plates.
8. Pour the pear juice into glasses and serve alongside the baked chicken breasts.
9. Garnish the chicken with fresh parsley, if desired.

- Calories: 250 kcal
- Protein: 30g
- Fat: 10g
- Carbohydrates: 10g
- Fiber: 0g
- Sugar: 8g

Difficulty

Rating

10 Pineapple Gelatin Cup With Cottage Cheese

Introduction

Pineapple gelatin cups with cottage cheese are a refreshing and nourishing option for individuals in Stage 1 of diverticulitis recovery. This combination provides hydration, protein, and a hint of sweetness from the pineapple gelatin, making it easy on the digestive system.

Ingredients

- 1 package (0.3 oz) pineapple-flavored gelatin
- 1 cup hot water
- 1 cup cold water
- 1/2 cup cottage cheese
- Fresh pineapple chunks for garnish (optional)

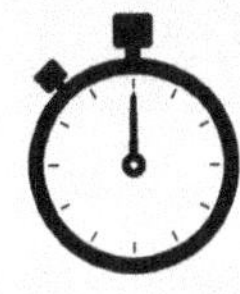 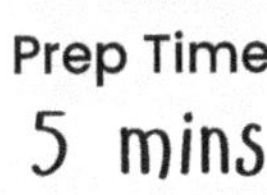
Prep Time
5 mins

Cook Time
2-3 hours
(chilling time)

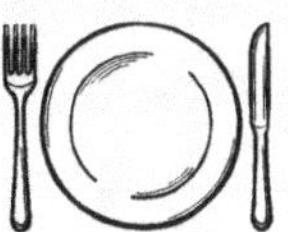
Serving
2

Preparation Method

1. In a mixing bowl, dissolve the pineapple-flavored gelatin in hot water, stirring until completely dissolved.
2. Add-in the cold water and stir until thoroughly mixed.
3. Divide the gelatin mixture among serving cups or molds.
4. Refrigerate for 2-3 hours or until the gelatin is set.
5. Once the gelatin is set, top each cup with a dollop of cottage cheese.
6. Garnish with fresh pineapple chunks, if desired.
7. Serve the pineapple gelatin cups with cottage cheese chilled.

- Calories: 120 kcal
- Protein: 8g
- Fat: 2g
- Carbohydrates: 20g
- Fiber: 0g
- Sugar: 16g

Difficulty

Rating

STAGE 2: HEALING AND STABILIZATION RECIPE

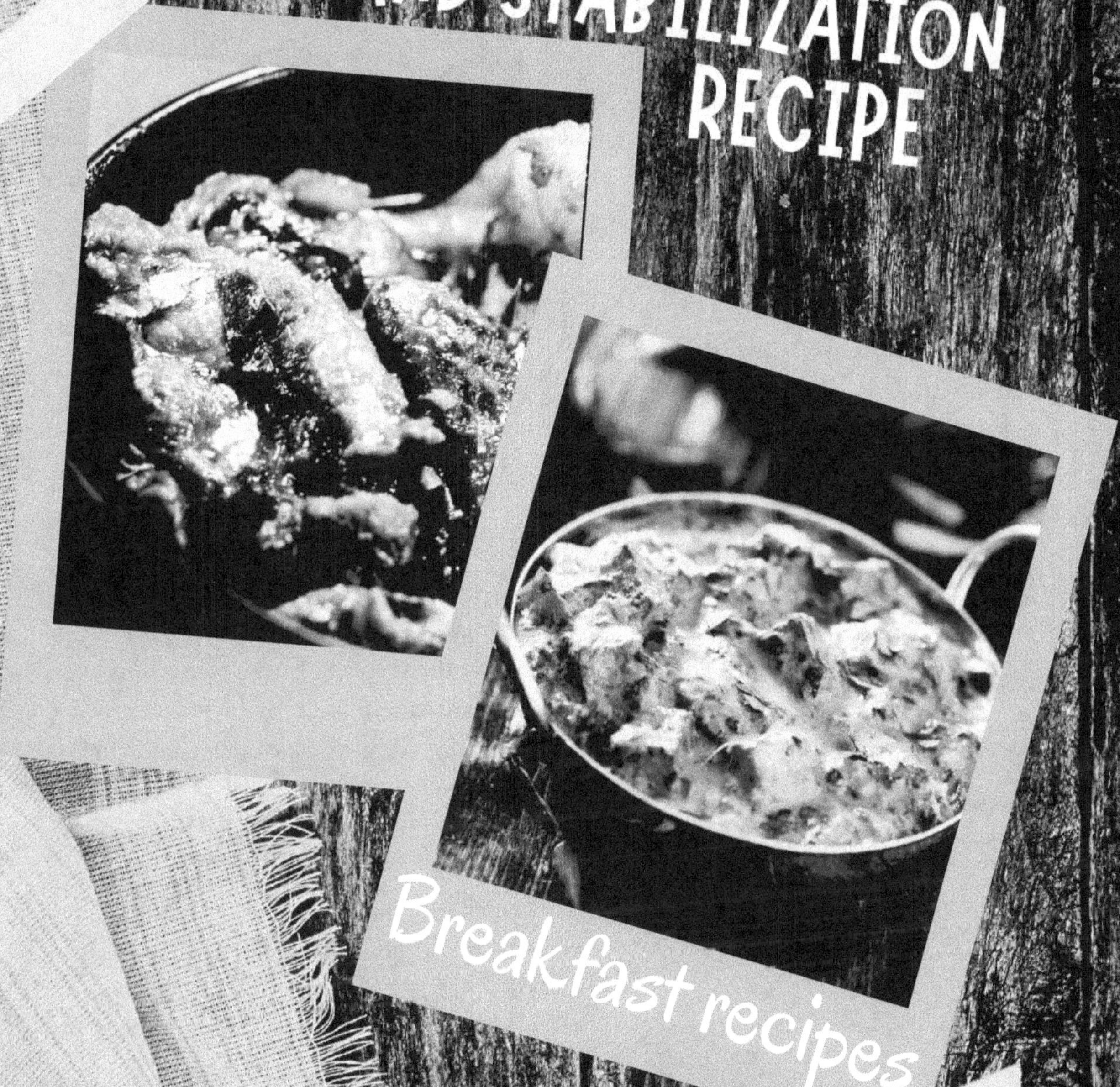

Breakfast recipes

Prep Time

Cook Time

Rating

Difficulty

Instructions

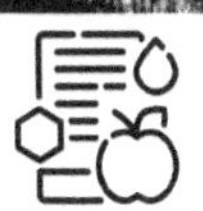
Nutritional Value

Serving

Oatmeal
With Mashed Banana

Introduction

Oatmeal with mashed banana is a wholesome and comforting option for individuals in Stage 2 of diverticulitis healing and stabilization. This breakfast provides a blend of soluble fiber from the oatmeal and potassium-rich mashed banana, promoting digestive health and overall well-being.

Ingredients

- 1/2 cup rolled oats
- 1 cup water or milk of choice
- 1 ripe banana, mashed
- Cinnamon or honey for optional sweetness
- Sliced almonds or walnuts for garnish (optional)

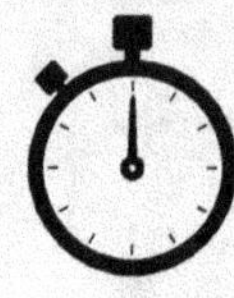   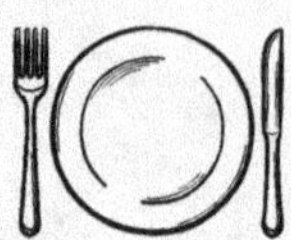

Prep Time	Cook Time	Serving
2 mins	5-7 mins	1

Preparation Method

1. In a small saucepan, bring the water or milk to a gentle boil over medium heat.
2. Add and stir-in the rolled oats, then turn down the heat.
3. Simmer the oats, stirring occasionally, for 5-7 minutes or until thickened to your desired consistency.
4. Remove the saucepan from the heat and stir in the mashed banana until well combined.
5. Optionally, add a sprinkle of cinnamon or honey for sweetness.
6. Divide the oatmeal with mashed banana among serving bowls.
7. Garnish with sliced almonds or walnuts, if desired.
8. Serve the oatmeal with mashed banana warm.

- Calories: 250 kcal
- Protein: 6g
- Fat: 3g
- Carbohydrates: 50g
- Fiber: 6g
- Sugar: 15g

Difficulty

Rating

2 Scrambled Eggs With Spinach

Introduction

Scrambled eggs with spinach is a nutritious and satisfying option for individuals in Stage 2 of diverticulitis healing and stabilization. This protein-rich breakfast combines the gentle texture of scrambled eggs with the added benefits of spinach, promoting digestive health and providing essential nutrients.

Ingredients

- 2 eggs
- 1 cup fresh spinach leaves, chopped
- Salt and pepper to taste
- Olive oil or butter for cooking
- Fresh parsley for garnish (optional)

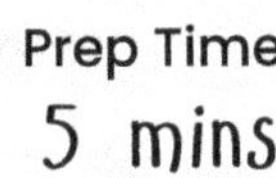

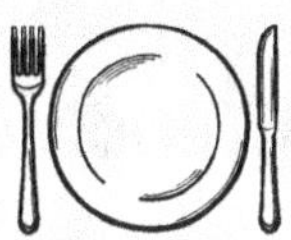

Prep Time
5 mins

Cook Time
5 mins

Serving
1

Preparation Method

1. Crack the eggs into a bowl and whisk until well beaten.
2. Heat a non-stick skillet over medium heat and add a drizzle of olive oil or a pat of butter.
3. Once the skillet is hot, add the chopped spinach and sauté for 1-2 minutes until wilted.
4. Pour the beaten eggs into the skillet over the wilted spinach.
5. Gently stir the eggs and spinach together, cooking until the eggs are scrambled and cooked through.
6. Season with salt and pepper to your preferred taste.
7. Transfer the scrambled eggs with spinach to a serving plate.
8. Garnish with fresh parsley, if desired.
9. Serve the scrambled eggs with spinach hot.

- Calories: 200 kcal
- Protein: 12g
- Fat: 15g
- Carbohydrates: 5g
- Fiber: 2g
- Sugar: 1g

Difficulty

Rating

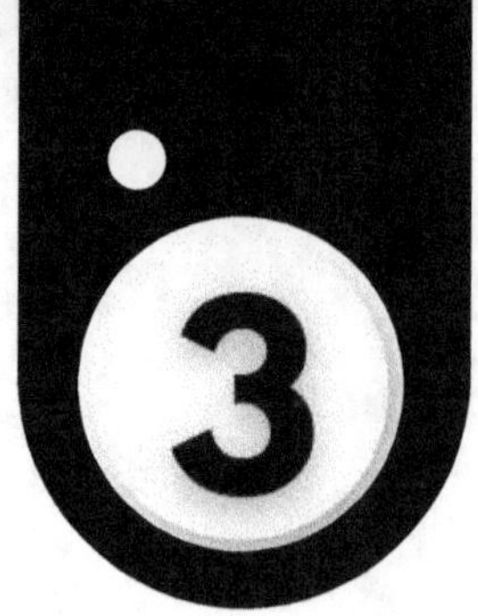

Greek Yogurt Parfait

Introduction

Greek yogurt parfait is a delicious and nutritious option for individuals in Stage 2 of diverticulitis healing and stabilization. This breakfast combines creamy Greek yogurt with fresh fruit and crunchy granola, providing a balance of protein, fiber, and essential nutrients to support digestive health

Ingredients

- 1 cup Greek yogurt
- 1/2 cup fresh berries (such as strawberries, blueberries, or raspberries)
- 1/4 cup granola
- Honey or maple syrup for optional sweetness
- Fresh mint leaves for garnish (optional)

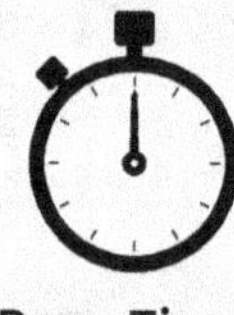 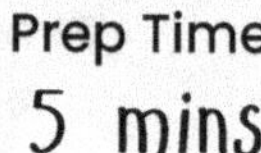  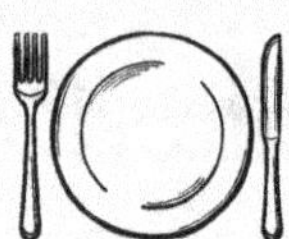

Prep Time	Cook Time	Serving
5 mins	0 mins	1

Preparation Method

1. In a serving glass or bowl, layer the Greek yogurt, fresh berries, and granola.
2. Drizzle with honey or maple syrup for sweetness, if desired.
3. Repeat the layers until the glass or bowl is filled, ending with a sprinkle of granola on top.
4. Garnish with fresh mint leaves, if desired.
5. Serve the Greek yogurt parfait immediately.

- Calories: 300 kcal
- Protein: 20g
- Fat: 10g
- Carbohydrates: 35g
- Fiber: 5g
- Sugar: 15g

Difficulty

Rating

4 Whole Grain Toast With *Avocado*

Introduction

Whole grain toast with avocado is a satisfying and nutritious option for individuals in Stage 2 of diverticulitis healing and stabilization. This breakfast provides fiber-rich whole grains and healthy fats from avocado, promoting digestive health and supporting overall well-being.

Ingredients

- 2 slices whole grain bread
- 1 ripe avocado
- Salt and pepper to taste
- Red pepper flakes or sliced tomatoes for optional garnish
- Fresh cilantro or parsley for garnish (optional)

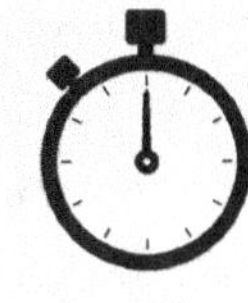 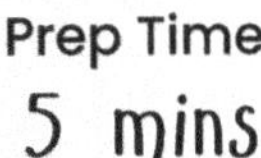  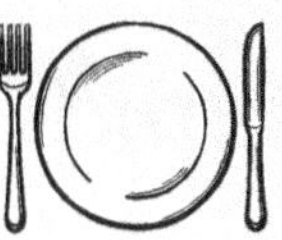

Prep Time 5 mins **Cook Time** 5 mins **Serving** 1

Preparation Method

1. Toast the whole grain bread slices until golden brown and crisp.
2. Meanwhile, halve the avocado and remove the pit.
3. Scoop the avocado flesh into a bowl and mash it with a fork until smooth.
4. Season the mashed avocado with salt and pepper to taste.
5. Spread the mashed avocado evenly onto the toasted bread slices.
6. Optionally, garnish with a sprinkle of red pepper flakes or sliced tomatoes for extra flavor and color.
7. Garnish with fresh cilantro or parsley, if desired.
8. Serve the whole grain toast with avocado immediately.

- Calories: 300 kcal
- Protein: 8g
- Fat: 15g
- Carbohydrates: 35g
- Fiber: 10g
- Sugar: 3g

Difficulty

Rating

Smoothie Bowl

Introduction

A smoothie bowl is a refreshing and nutrient-packed option for individuals in Stage 2 of diverticulitis healing and stabilization. This breakfast combines blended fruits and vegetables with toppings like nuts, seeds, and granola, providing essential vitamins, minerals, and fiber to support digestive health and overall well-being.

Ingredients

- 1 ripe banana, frozen
- 1/2 cup frozen berries (such as strawberries, blueberries, or raspberries)
- 1/2 cup spinach or kale leaves
- 1/2 cup Greek yogurt
- 1/4 cup almond milk or other milk of choice
- Toppings: sliced fresh fruit, granola, chia seeds, shredded coconut, nuts, seeds, etc.

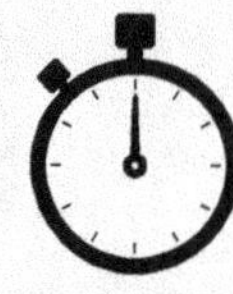 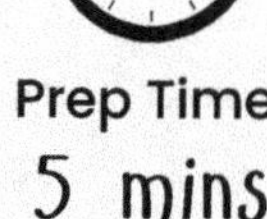  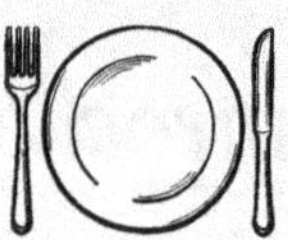

Prep Time 5 mins

Cook Time 0 mins

Serving 1

Preparation Method

1. In a blender, combine the frozen banana, frozen berries, spinach or kale leaves, Greek yogurt, and almond milk.
2. Blend until smooth and creamy, adding more almond milk if needed to reach desired consistency.
3. Pour the smoothie into a bowl.
4. Arrange your choice of toppings on top of the smoothie.
5. Serve the smoothie bowl immediately with a spoon.

- Calories: 250 kcal
- Protein: 15g
- Fat: 5g
- Carbohydrates: 40g
- Fiber: 8g
- Sugar: 20g

Difficulty

Rating

Chia Seed Pudding

Introduction

Chia seed pudding is a nutritious and versatile option for individuals in Stage 2 of diverticulitis healing and stabilization. This pudding is made by soaking chia seeds in liquid until they form a thick, pudding-like consistency, providing a good source of fiber, omega-3 fatty acids, and antioxidants to support digestive health and overall well-being.

Ingredients

- 2 tablespoons chia seeds
- 1/2 cup almond milk or other milk of choice
- 1/2 teaspoon vanilla extract
- Optional sweeteners: honey, maple syrup, or stevia
- Toppings: sliced fresh fruit, nuts, seeds, shredded coconut, etc.

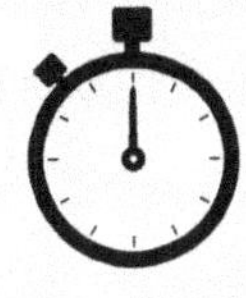  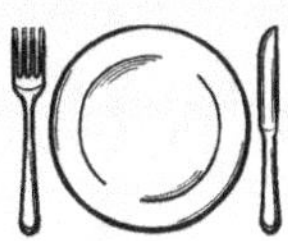

Prep Time
5 mins
(Plus chilling time)

Cook Time
0 mins

Serving
1

Preparation Method

1. In a bowl, combine the chia seeds, almond milk, and vanilla extract.
2. Stir well to combine.
3. Optionally, sweeten the mixture with your choice of sweetener to taste.
4. Cover the bowl and refrigerate for at least 2 hours or overnight, stirring occasionally to prevent clumping.
5. Once the chia seeds have absorbed the liquid and formed a thick pudding consistency, give the pudding a final stir.
6. Divide the chia seed pudding into serving bowls.
7. Top with your choice of toppings, such as sliced fresh fruit, nuts, seeds, or shredded coconut.
8. Serve the chia seed pudding chilled.

- Calories: 150 kcal
- Protein: 5g
- Fat: 8g
- Carbohydrates: 15g
- Fiber: 8g
- Sugar: 0g

Difficulty

Rating

Vegetable Frittata

Introduction

A vegetable frittata is a flavorful and nutritious option for individuals in Stage 2 of diverticulitis healing and stabilization. This dish combines eggs with an assortment of vegetables, providing protein, fiber, and essential vitamins and minerals to support digestive health and overall well-being.

Ingredients

- 4 large eggs
- 1/4 cup milk (any type)
- Salt and pepper to taste
- 1 tablespoon olive oil
- 1/2 small onion, diced
- 1 bell pepper, diced
- 1 cup spinach leaves, chopped
- 1/2 cup cherry tomatoes, halved
- 1/4 cup shredded cheese (optional)
- Fresh herbs for garnish (optional)

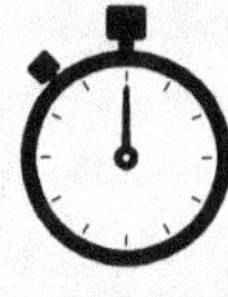  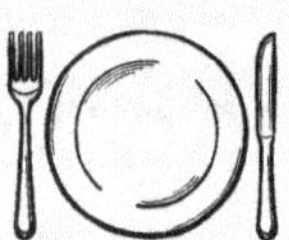

Prep Time 10 mins **Cook Time** 20 mins **Serving** 2-4

Preparation Method

1. Preheat the oven to 350°F (175°C).
2. Whisk the eggs, milk, salt, and pepper in a mixing bowl until they're thoroughly combined. Set aside.
3. The olive oil should be heated up over medium heat, using an oven-safe skillet.
4. Add the diced onion and bell pepper to the skillet and sauté until softened, about 3-4 minutes.
5. Add the chopped spinach leaves and cherry tomatoes to the skillet and cook for an additional 1-2 minutes until the spinach wilts.
6. Pour the egg mixture evenly over the vegetables in the skillet.
7. Sprinkle shredded cheese on top, if using.
8. Transfer the skillet to the preheated oven and bake for 12-15 minutes or until the frittata is set and slightly golden on top.
9. Remove the skillet from the oven and let the frittata cool for a few minutes.
10. Slice the frittata into wedges and garnish with fresh herbs, if desired.
11. Serve the vegetable frittata warm or at room temperature.

- Calories: 150 kcal
- Protein: 8g
- Fat: 10g
- Carbohydrates: 6g
- Fiber: 2g
- Sugar: 3g

Difficulty

Rating

8 Whole Grain Pancakes

Introduction

Whole grain pancakes are a delicious and wholesome option for individuals in Stage 2 of diverticulitis healing and stabilization. These pancakes are made with whole grain flour and can be topped with fresh fruit and a drizzle of honey or maple syrup for added flavor and sweetness.

Ingredients

- 1 cup whole wheat flour
- 1 tablespoon baking powder
- 1/4 teaspoon salt
- 1 tablespoon honey or maple syrup
- 1 cup milk (any type)
- 1 large egg
- 2 tablespoons melted butter or oil
- Optional toppings: fresh fruit, Greek yogurt, honey, maple syrup, etc.

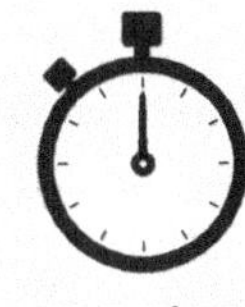  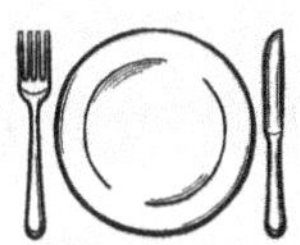

Prep Time
10 mins

Cook Time
15 mins

Serving
8-10 pancakes

Preparation Method

1. Mix the whole wheat flour, baking powder, and salt in a sizable mixing bowl.
2. In a separate bowl, whisk together the honey or maple syrup, milk, egg, and melted butter or oil until well combined.
3. Add in the wet ingredients into the dry ingredients and stir/mix until they're well blended. Do not overmix; lumps are okay.
4. Heat a non-stick skillet or griddle over medium heat and lightly grease with butter or oil.
5. For every pancake, transfer roughly 1/4 cup of batter onto the skillet.
6. Cook the pancakes for 2-3 minutes on one side, or until bubbles form on the surface and the edges start to set.
7. Flip the pancakes and cook for another 1-2 minutes on the other side, or until golden brown and fully cooked.
8. After the pancakes are done, transfer them to a platter and continue the process with the remaining batter.
9. Serve the whole grain pancakes warm with your choice of toppings, such as fresh fruit, Greek yogurt, honey, or maple syrup.

- Calories: 100 kcal
- Protein: 4g
- Fat: 3g
- Carbohydrates: 15g
- Fiber: 2g
- Sugar: 3g

Difficulty

Rating

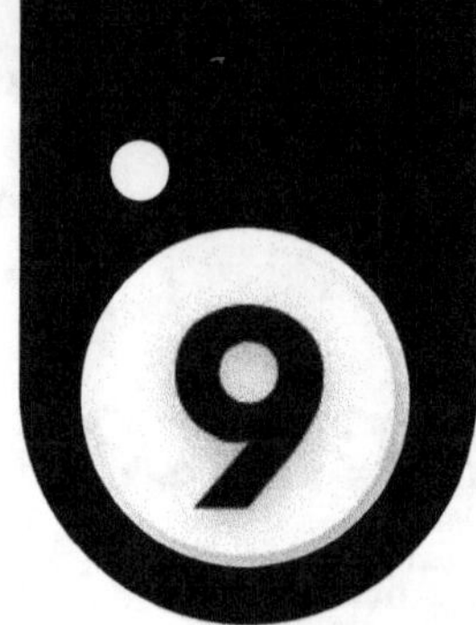

Quinoa Breakfast Bowl

Introduction

A quinoa breakfast bowl is a nutritious and satisfying option for individuals in Stage 2 of diverticulitis healing and stabilization. This breakfast combines cooked quinoa with nutrient-rich toppings like fresh fruit, nuts, seeds, and Greek yogurt, providing a balance of protein, fiber, and essential vitamins and minerals to support digestive health and overall well-being.

Ingredients

- 1/2 cup quinoa, rinsed
- 1 cup water or vegetable broth
- 1/2 cup Greek yogurt
- 1/2 cup mixed berries (such as strawberries, blueberries, or raspberries)
- 1/4 cup sliced almonds or chopped walnuts
- 1 tablespoon honey or maple syrup
- Fresh mint leaves for garnish (optional)

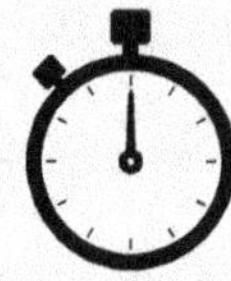
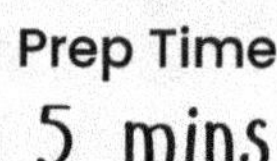

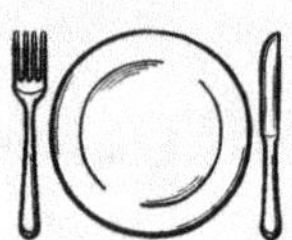

Prep Time
5 mins

Cook Time
20 mins

Serving
2

Preparation Method

1. In a small saucepan, combine the quinoa and water or vegetable broth.
2. Bring to a boil, then reduce the heat to low and simmer, covered, for 15-20 minutes or until the quinoa is tender and the liquid is absorbed.
3. Fluff the cooked quinoa with a fork and divide it into serving bowls.
4. Top each bowl of quinoa with Greek yogurt, mixed berries, sliced almonds or chopped walnuts, and a drizzle of honey or maple syrup.
5. If preferred you can garnish with fresh mint leaves.
6. Serve the quinoa breakfast bowls warm or chilled.

- Calories: 300 kcal
- Protein: 15g
- Fat: 10g
- Carbohydrates: 40g
- Fiber: 6g
- Sugar: 15g

Difficulty

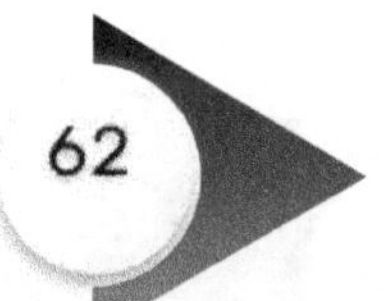

Rating

Breakfast Burrito

Introduction

A breakfast burrito is a delicious and convenient option for individuals in Stage 2 of diverticulitis healing and stabilization. This breakfast combines scrambled eggs with sautéed vegetables and cheese, wrapped in a whole grain tortilla, providing protein, fiber, and essential nutrients to support digestive health and overall well-being.

Ingredients

- 2 large eggs, beaten
- 1/4 cup diced onion
- 1/4 cup diced bell pepper
- 1/4 cup diced tomato
- 1/4 cup shredded cheese (such as cheddar or Monterey Jack)
- 2 whole grain tortillas
- Salt and pepper to taste
- Salsa, avocado, or Greek yogurt for optional garnish

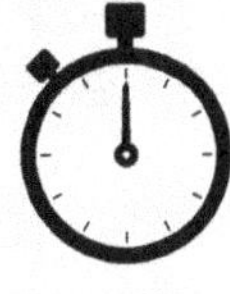  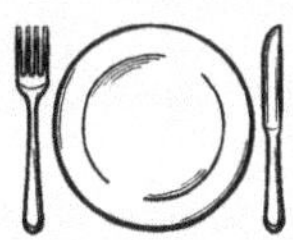

Prep Time 10 mins

Cook Time 10 mins

Serving 2

Preparation Method

1. In a skillet, heat a drizzle of olive oil over medium heat.
2. Add the diced onion and bell pepper to the skillet and sauté until softened, about 3-4 minutes.
3. Add the diced tomato to the skillet and cook for an additional 1-2 minutes.
4. Spoon the veggies to one half of the skillet and transfer the beaten eggs to the other half.
5. Cook the eggs, stirring occasionally, until scrambled and cooked through.
6. Season the scrambled eggs and vegetables with salt and pepper to taste.
7. Warm the whole grain tortillas in the microwave or on a skillet for a few seconds.
8. Divide the scrambled eggs and vegetables evenly between the tortillas.
9. Sprinkle shredded cheese on top of the eggs and vegetables.
10. Roll up the tortillas into burritos, folding in the sides as you go.
11. Optionally, garnish the breakfast burritos with salsa, avocado, or Greek yogurt.
12. Serve the breakfast burritos immediately.

- Calories: 350 kcal
- Protein: 15g
- Fat: 15g
- Carbohydrates: 30g
- Fiber: 5g
- Sugar: 5g

Difficulty

Rating

STAGE 2: HEALING AND STABILIZATION RECIPE

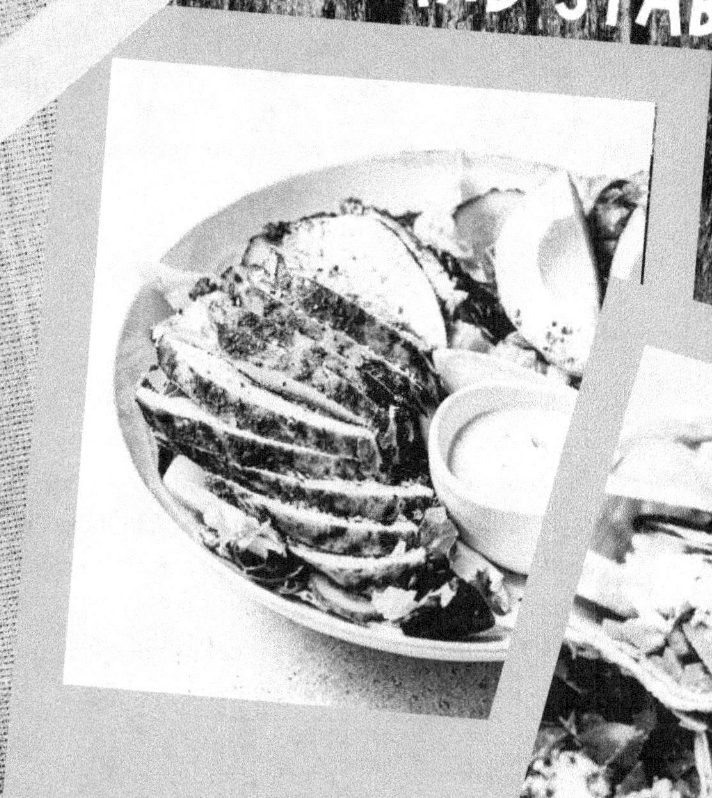

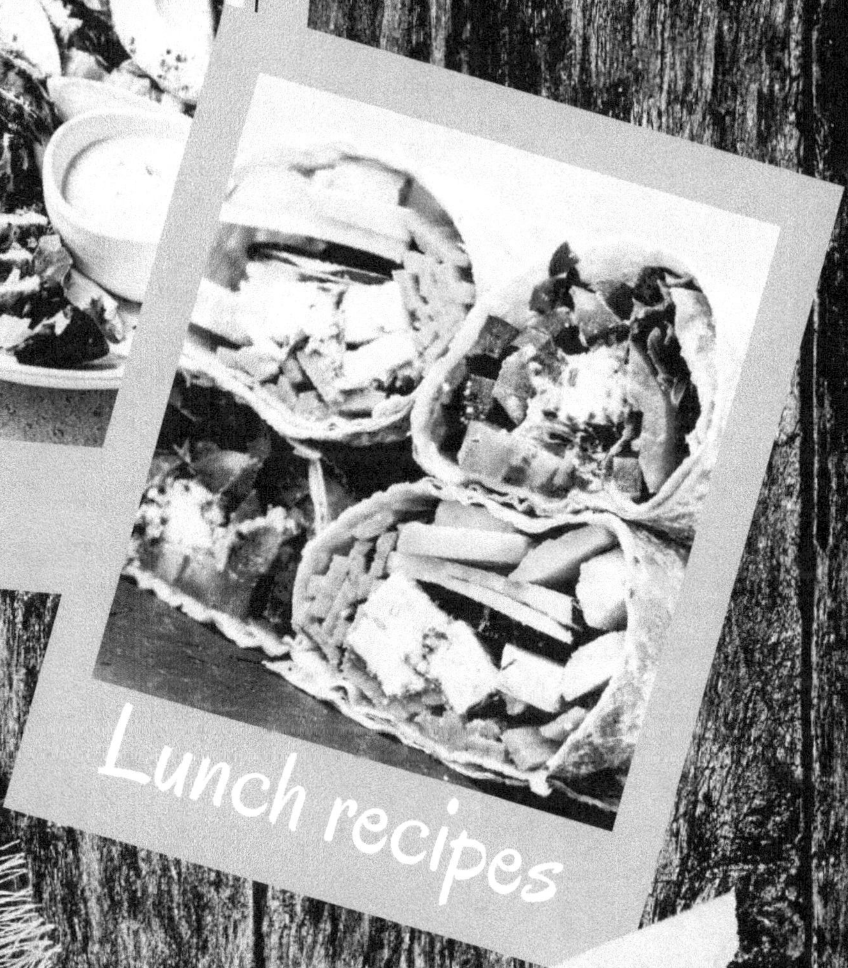

Lunch recipes

Prep Time

Cook Time

Rating

Difficulty

Instructions

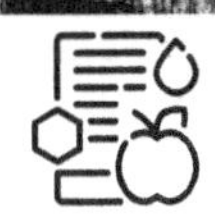

Nutritional Value

Serving

Grilled Chicken Salad

Introduction

A grilled chicken salad is a nutritious and satisfying option for individuals in Stage 2 of diverticulitis healing and stabilization. This salad combines lean protein from grilled chicken with an assortment of fresh vegetables and a flavorful dressing, providing essential nutrients to support digestive health and overall well-being.

Ingredients

- 2 boneless, skinless chicken breasts
- Salt and pepper to taste
- 4 cups mixed salad greens (such as lettuce, spinach, or arugula)
- 1 cup cherry tomatoes, halved
- 1 cucumber, sliced
- 1/4 red onion, thinly sliced
- 1/4 cup sliced almonds or chopped walnuts
- Optional toppings: avocado slices, crumbled feta cheese, dried cranberries, etc.

For the dressing:
- 2 tablespoons extra virgin olive oil
- 1 tablespoon balsamic vinegar
- 1 teaspoon Dijon mustard
- Salt and pepper to taste

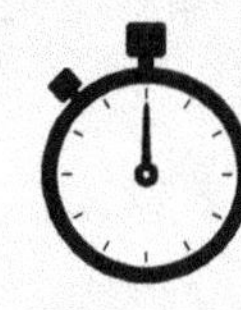   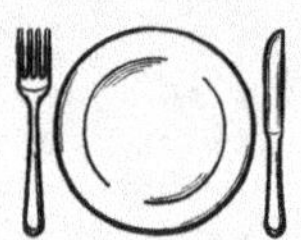

Prep Time	Cook Time	Serving
10 mins	15 mins	2

Preparation Method

1. Preheat your grill pan or grill over medium-high heat.
2. Season the chicken breasts with salt and pepper.
3. Grill the chicken breasts for 5-7 minutes per side, or until cooked through and no longer pink in the center.
4. Remove the chicken from the grill and let it rest for a few minutes before slicing.
5. In a large salad bowl, combine the mixed salad greens, cherry tomatoes, cucumber, red onion, and sliced almonds or chopped walnuts.
6. In a small bowl, whisk together the extra virgin olive oil, balsamic vinegar, Dijon mustard, salt, and pepper to make the dressing.
7. Drizzle the dressing over the salad and toss to coat evenly.
8. Divide the salad onto plates and top each portion with sliced grilled chicken.
9. Add optional toppings like avocado slices, crumbled feta cheese, or dried cranberries, if desired.
10. Serve the grilled chicken salad immediately.

- Calories: 300 kcal
- Protein: 25g
- Fat: 15g
- Carbohydrates: 15g
- Fiber: 5g
- Sugar: 5g

Difficulty

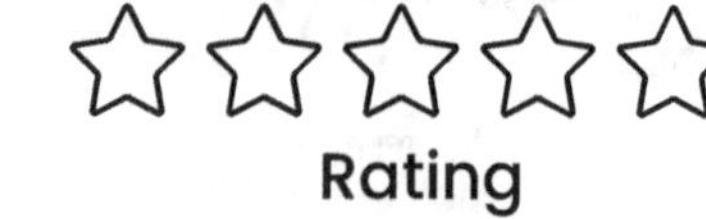

Rating

Lentil Soup

Introduction

Lentil soup is a hearty and nourishing option for individuals in Stage 2 of diverticulitis healing and stabilization. This soup combines fiber-rich lentils with vegetables and flavorful seasonings, providing protein, fiber, and essential nutrients to support digestive health and overall well-being.

Ingredients

- 1 cup dried green or brown lentils, rinsed
- 4 cups vegetable broth
- 1 tablespoon olive oil
- 1 onion, diced
- 2 carrots, diced
- 2 celery stalks, diced
- 2 cloves garlic, minced
- 1 teaspoon ground cumin
- 1 teaspoon ground coriander
- 1/2 teaspoon smoked paprika
- Salt and pepper to taste
- Fresh parsley for garnish (optional)

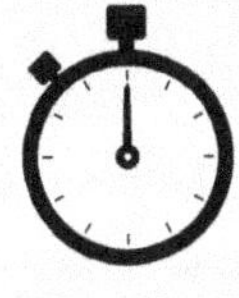  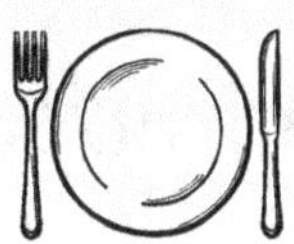

Prep Time	Cook Time	Serving
10 mins	30 mins	4

Preparation Method

1. In a large pot, heat the olive oil over medium heat.
2. Add the diced onion, carrots, and celery to the pot and sauté until softened, about 5 minutes.
3. Add the minced garlic, ground cumin, ground coriander, and smoked paprika to the pot. Cook for a another 1-2 minutes, until fragrant/aromatic.
4. Add the rinsed lentils and vegetable broth to the pot. Stir to combine.
5. Bring the soup to a boil, then reduce the heat to low and simmer, covered, for 20-25 minutes or until the lentils are tender.
6. Season the soup with salt and pepper to your preferred taste.
7. If desired, use an immersion blender to partially blend the soup for a smoother consistency.
8. Ladle the lentil soup into bowls and garnish with fresh parsley, if using.
9. Serve the lentil soup hot.

- Calories: 250 kcal
- Protein: 15g
- Fat: 5g
- Carbohydrates: 40g
- Fiber: 15g
- Sugar: 5g

Difficulty

Rating

Quinoa Salad

Introduction

Quinoa salad is a nutritious and flavorful option for individuals in Stage 2 of diverticulitis healing and stabilization. This salad combines protein-packed quinoa with an array of colorful vegetables and a zesty dressing, providing essential nutrients to support digestive health and overall well-being.

Ingredients

- 1 cup quinoa, rinsed
- 2 cups water or vegetable broth
- 1 cucumber, diced
- 1 bell pepper, diced
- 1 cup cherry tomatoes, halved
- 1/4 red onion, thinly sliced
- 1/4 cup chopped fresh parsley
- 1/4 cup crumbled feta cheese (optional)

For the dressing:

- 3 tablespoons extra virgin olive oil
- 2 tablespoons lemon juice
- 1 teaspoon Dijon mustard
- 1 clove garlic, minced
- Salt and pepper to taste

  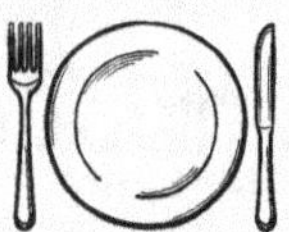

Prep Time 10 mins

Cook Time 20 mins

Serving 4

Preparation Method

1. In a medium saucepan, combine the quinoa and water or vegetable broth.
2. Bring to a boil, then reduce the heat to low and simmer, covered, for 15-20 minutes or until the quinoa is tender and the liquid is absorbed.
3. Fluff the cooked quinoa with a fork and let it cool slightly.
4. In a large salad bowl, combine the cooked quinoa, diced cucumber, bell pepper, cherry tomatoes, red onion, and chopped fresh parsley.
5. In a small bowl, whisk together the extra virgin olive oil, lemon juice, Dijon mustard, minced garlic, salt, and pepper to make the dressing.
6. Pour the dressing over the quinoa salad and toss to coat evenly.
7. If using, sprinkle crumbled feta cheese over the salad.
8. Serve the quinoa salad immediately, or refrigerate for later use.

- Calories: 250 kcal
- Protein: 7g
- Fat: 10g
- Carbohydrates: 35g
- Fiber: 5g
- Sugar: 3g

Difficulty

Rating

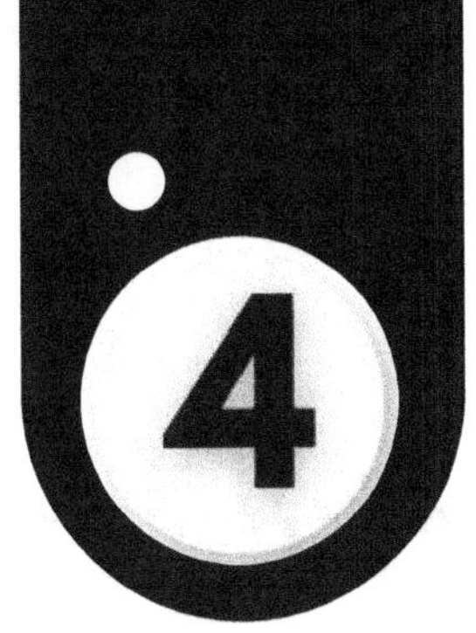

Turkey and Vegetable Stir-Fry

Introduction

Turkey and vegetable stir-fry is a quick and nutritious option for individuals in Stage 2 of diverticulitis healing and stabilization. This dish combines lean turkey breast with an assortment of colorful vegetables and savory seasonings, providing protein, fiber, and essential nutrients to support digestive health and overall well-being.

Ingredients

- 1 tablespoon olive oil
- 1 pound turkey breast, thinly sliced
- Salt and pepper to taste
- 1 bell pepper, thinly sliced
- 1 cup broccoli florets
- 1 cup snap peas or sugar snap peas
- 2 cloves garlic, minced
- 2 tablespoons low-sodium soy sauce
- 1 tablespoon honey or maple syrup
- 1 teaspoon cornstarch (optional, for thickening)
- Cooked brown rice or quinoa, for serving

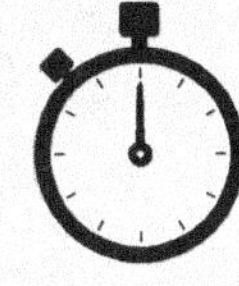  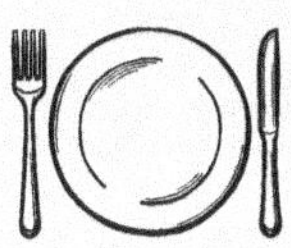

Prep Time 15 mins

Cook Time 15 mins

Serving 4

Preparation Method

1. The olive oil should be heated up over medium heat, using a large skillet or wok.
2. Season the thinly sliced turkey breast with salt and pepper.
3. Add the turkey breast to the skillet and cook for 3-4 minutes, stirring occasionally, until browned and cooked through.
4. Remove the cooked turkey from the skillet and set aside.
5. In the same skillet, add the sliced bell pepper, broccoli florets, snap peas, and minced garlic.
6. Stir-fry the vegetables for 3-4 minutes, or until crisp-tender.
7. Return the cooked turkey to the skillet with the vegetables.
8. In a small bowl, whisk together the low-sodium soy sauce, honey or maple syrup, and cornstarch (if using).
9. Pour the sauce over the turkey and vegetables in the skillet.
10. Cook for an additional 1-2 minutes, stirring constantly, until the sauce thickens and coats the turkey and vegetables evenly.
11. Remove the skillet from the heat.
12. Serve the turkey and vegetable stir-fry hot over cooked brown rice or quinoa.

- Calories: 200 kcal
- Protein: 25g
- Fat: 8g
- Carbohydrates: 10g
- Fiber: 3g
- Sugar: 5g

Difficulty

Rating

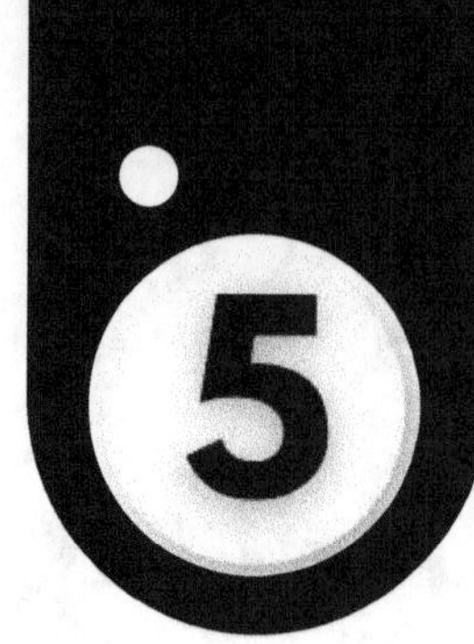

5 Baked Salmon With Steamed Vegetables

Introduction

Baked salmon with steamed vegetables is a wholesome and nutritious option for individuals in Stage 2 of diverticulitis healing and stabilization. This dish features omega-3 rich salmon fillets baked to perfection and served alongside a colorful assortment of steamed vegetables, providing a balanced combination of protein, fiber, and essential nutrients to support digestive health and overall well-being.

Ingredients

- 2 salmon fillets
- Salt and pepper to taste
- 2 cups mixed vegetables (such as broccoli, carrots, and bell peppers), cut into bite-sized pieces
- 1 tablespoon olive oil
- 1 tablespoon lemon juice
- 1 teaspoon minced garlic
- 1 teaspoon dried herbs (such as thyme, rosemary, or dill)
- Lemon wedges for garnish (optional)

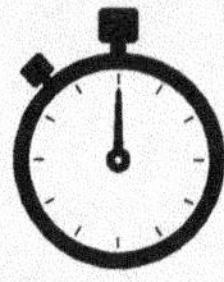

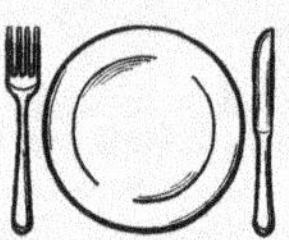

Prep Time	Cook Time	Serving
10 mins	15 mins	2

Preparation Method

1. Preheat the oven to 375°F (190°C).
2. Place the salmon fillets on a baking sheet lined with parchment paper.
3. Season the salmon fillets with salt and pepper to your preferred taste.
4. In a small bowl, whisk together the olive oil, lemon juice, minced garlic, and dried herbs.
5. Brush the olive oil mixture over the salmon fillets.
6. Arrange the mixed vegetables around the salmon fillets on the baking sheet.
7. Drizzle any remaining olive oil mixture over the vegetables.
8. Bake in the preheated oven for 12-15 minutes, or until the salmon is cooked through and flakes easily with a fork.
9. While the salmon is baking, steam the mixed vegetables until tender, about 5-7 minutes.
10. Remove the baked salmon and steamed vegetables from the oven and let them cool slightly.
11. Serve the baked salmon alongside the steamed vegetables.
12. Garnish with lemon wedges, if desired.
13. Enjoy the baked salmon with steamed vegetables hot.

- Calories: 300 kcal
- Protein: 25g
- Fat: 15g
- Carbohydrates: 15g
- Fiber: 5g
- Sugar: 5g

Difficulty

Rating

Chickpea Salad

Introduction

Chickpea salad is a vibrant and satisfying option for individuals in Stage 2 of diverticulitis healing and stabilization. This salad features protein-packed chickpeas tossed with an array of colorful vegetables and a tangy vinaigrette dressing, providing a nutritious and flavorful meal to support digestive health and overall well-being.

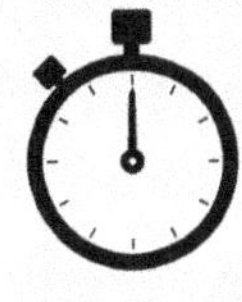

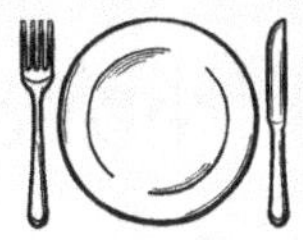

Prep Time — 10 mins

Cook Time — 30 mins

Serving — 4

Preparation Method

1. In a large salad bowl, combine the chickpeas, cherry tomatoes, cucumber, bell pepper, red onion, and chopped fresh parsley.
2. In a small bowl, whisk together the extra virgin olive oil, red wine vinegar, Dijon mustard, salt, and pepper to make the vinaigrette dressing.
3. Pour the dressing over the chickpea salad and toss to coat evenly.
4. Let the chickpea salad marinate in the refrigerator for at least 30 minutes to allow the flavors to meld together.
5. Serve the chickpea salad chilled as a refreshing and nutritious meal option.

Ingredients

- 1 can (15 ounces) chickpeas, drained and rinsed
- 1 cup cherry tomatoes, halved
- 1 cucumber, diced
- 1 bell pepper, diced
- 1/4 red onion, thinly sliced
- 1/4 cup chopped fresh parsley
- 2 tablespoons extra virgin olive oil
- 1 tablespoon red wine vinegar
- 1 teaspoon Dijon mustard
- Salt and pepper to taste

- Calories: 200 kcal
- Protein: 8g
- Fat: 8g
- Carbohydrates: 25g
- Fiber: 6g
- Sugar: 5g

Difficulty

Rating

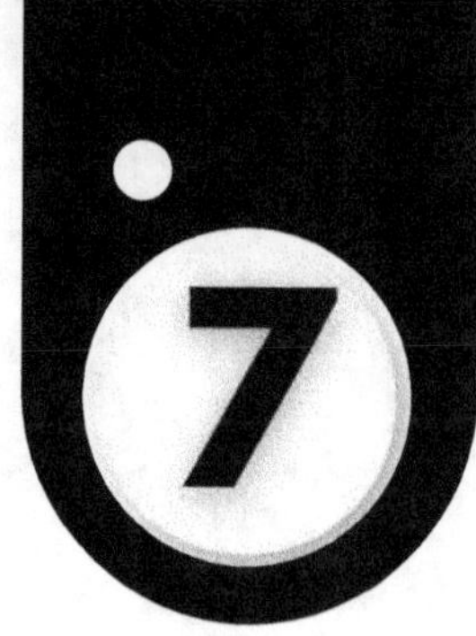

Tuna Stuffed Bell Peppers

Introduction

Tuna stuffed bell peppers are a delicious and nutritious option for individuals in Stage 2 of diverticulitis healing and stabilization. This dish features bell peppers filled with a savory mixture of tuna, vegetables, and herbs, providing protein, fiber, and essential nutrients to support digestive health and overall well-being.

Ingredients

- 4 bell peppers (any color), halved and seeds removed
- 2 cans (5 ounces each) tuna, drained
- 1/2 cup diced celery
- 1/2 cup diced cucumber
- 1/4 cup diced red onion
- 1/4 cup chopped fresh parsley
- 2 tablespoons lemon juice
- 2 tablespoons olive oil
- 1 teaspoon Dijon mustard
- Salt and pepper to taste
- Optional toppings: shredded cheese, chopped tomatoes, sliced olives

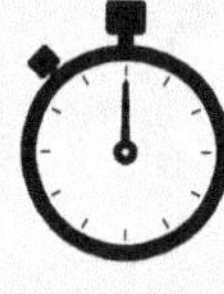  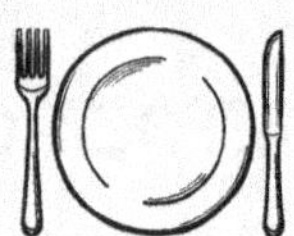

Prep Time 15 mins   **Cook Time** 30 mins   **Serving** 4

Preparation Method

1. Preheat the oven to 375°F (190°C).
2. Place the bell pepper halves in a baking dish, cut side up.
3. In a large mixing bowl, combine the drained tuna, diced celery, diced cucumber, diced red onion, chopped fresh parsley, lemon juice, olive oil, Dijon mustard, salt, and pepper. Mix well to combine.
4. Spoon the tuna mixture evenly into the bell pepper halves, pressing down gently to pack the filling.
5. Cover the baking dish with aluminum foil and bake in the preheated oven for 25-30 minutes, or until the bell peppers are tender.
6. Remove the foil and sprinkle optional toppings, if desired.
7. Return the stuffed bell peppers to the oven and bake for an additional 5 minutes, or until the toppings are heated through.
8. Remove from the oven and set aside to cool slightly before serving.
9. Serve the tuna stuffed bell peppers hot as a satisfying and nutritious meal option.

- Calories: 200 kcal
- Protein: 20g
- Fat: 8g
- Carbohydrates: 10g
- Fiber: 3g
- Sugar: 4g

Difficulty

Rating

Introduction

Veggie wrap is a flavorful and wholesome option for individuals in Stage 2 of diverticulitis healing and stabilization. This wrap features a whole grain tortilla filled with an assortment of colorful vegetables, creamy hummus, and tangy dressing, providing fiber, vitamins, and minerals to support digestive health and overall well-being.

Ingredients

- 4 whole grain tortillas
- 1 cup baby spinach leaves
- 1/2 cup shredded carrots
- 1/2 cup sliced cucumber
- 1/2 cup sliced bell peppers (any color)
- 1/4 cup sliced red onion
- 1/4 cup sliced olives (optional)
- 1/4 cup hummus
- 2 tablespoons balsamic vinaigrette or tahini dressing

Veggie Wrap

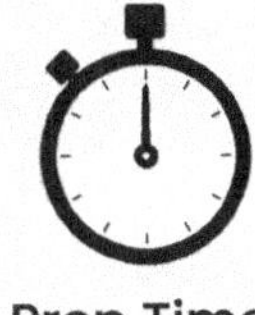

Prep Time
10 mins

Cook Time
0 mins

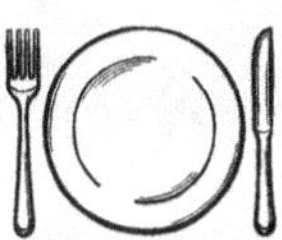

Serving
4

Preparation Method

1. Lay out the whole grain tortillas on a clean surface.
2. Spread a layer of hummus evenly over each tortilla.
3. Arrange the baby spinach leaves, shredded carrots, sliced cucumber, sliced bell peppers, sliced red onion, and sliced olives (if using) over the hummus on each tortilla.
4. Drizzle balsamic vinaigrette or tahini dressing over the vegetables.
5. Roll up each tortilla tightly to form a wrap.
6. Slice the veggie wraps in half diagonally.
7. Serve the veggie wraps immediately as a delicious and nutritious meal option.

- Calories: 250 kcal
- Protein: 8g
- Fat: 10g
- Carbohydrates: 30g
- Fiber: 6g
- Sugar: 4g

Difficulty

Rating

Introduction

Turkey and avocado wrap is a delicious and nutritious option for individuals in Stage 2 of diverticulitis healing and stabilization. This wrap features lean turkey breast, creamy avocado, and crunchy vegetables wrapped in a whole grain tortilla, providing protein, healthy fats, fiber, and essential nutrients to support digestive health and overall well-being.

Ingredients

- 4 whole grain tortillas
- 8 slices of cooked turkey breast
- 1 ripe avocado, thinly sliced
- 1 cup shredded lettuce
- 1/2 cup sliced cucumber
- 1/2 cup sliced bell peppers (any color)
- 1/4 cup sliced red onion
- 1/4 cup hummus or Greek yogurt
- Salt and pepper to taste

Turkey And Avocado Wrap

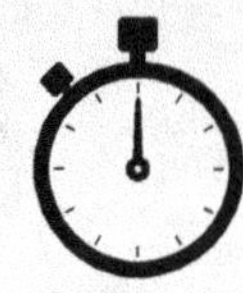
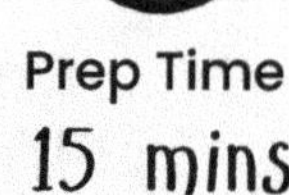

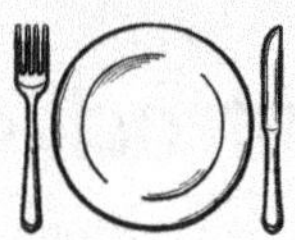

Prep Time
15 mins

Cook Time
0 mins

Serving
4

Preparation Method

1. Lay out the whole grain tortillas on a clean surface.
2. Spread a layer of hummus or Greek yogurt evenly over each tortilla.
3. Place 2 slices of cooked turkey breast on each tortilla.
4. Arrange the avocado slices, shredded lettuce, sliced cucumber, sliced bell peppers, and sliced red onion over the turkey on each tortilla.
5. Season with salt and pepper to taste.
6. Roll up each tortilla tightly to form a wrap.
7. Slice the turkey and avocado wraps in half diagonally.
8. Serve the wraps immediately as a satisfying and nutritious meal option.

- Calories: 300 kcal
- Protein: 20g
- Fat: 15g
- Carbohydrates: 25g
- Fiber: 8g
- Sugar: 4g

Difficulty

Rating

Egg Salad Lettuce Wraps

Introduction

Egg salad lettuce wraps are a light and refreshing option for individuals in Stage 2 of diverticulitis healing and stabilization. This recipe features creamy egg salad wrapped in crisp lettuce leaves, providing protein, healthy fats, and essential nutrients to support digestive health and overall well-being.

Ingredients

- 6 hard-boiled eggs, peeled and chopped
- 1/4 cup Greek yogurt or mayonnaise
- 1 tablespoon Dijon mustard
- 1 tablespoon chopped fresh dill (optional)
- Salt and pepper to taste
- 8 large lettuce leaves (such as romaine or butter lettuce)
- Optional toppings: sliced cherry tomatoes, sliced cucumbers, avocado slices

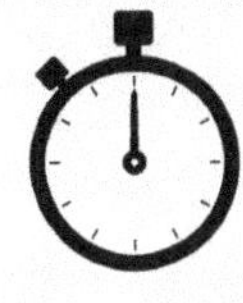  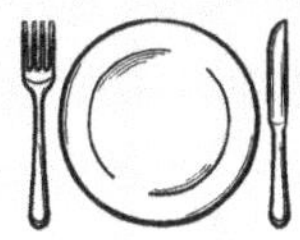

Prep Time 15 mins   **Cook Time** 0 mins   **Serving** 4

Preparation Method

1. In a mixing bowl, combine the chopped hard-boiled eggs, Greek yogurt or mayonnaise, Dijon mustard, chopped fresh dill (if using), salt, and pepper. Mix well to combine.
2. Lay out the large lettuce leaves on a clean surface.
3. Spoon the egg salad mixture onto each lettuce leaf.
4. Top with optional toppings such as sliced cherry tomatoes, sliced cucumbers, or avocado slices.
5. Roll up each lettuce leaf to form a wrap.
6. Serve the egg salad lettuce wraps immediately as a light and nutritious meal option.

- Calories: 180 kcal
- Protein: 12g
- Fat: 10g
- Carbohydrates: 6g
- Fiber: 2g
- Sugar: 2g

Difficulty

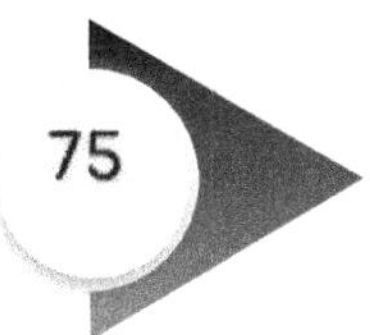

Rating

STAGE 2: HEALING AND STABILIZATION RECIPE

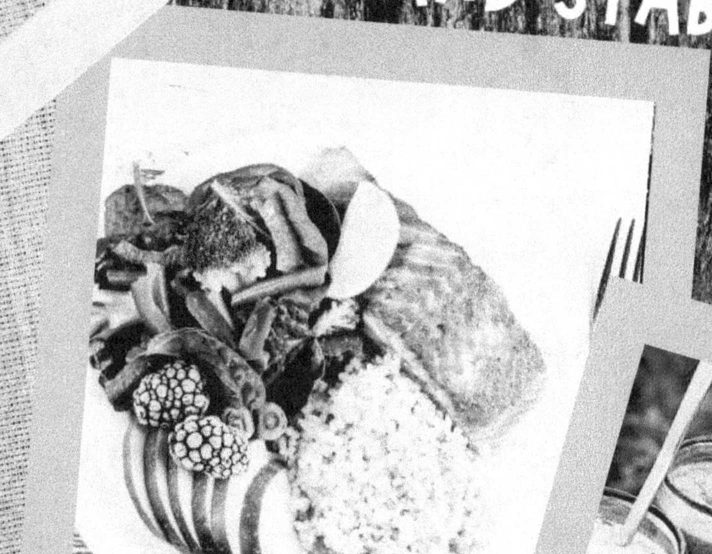

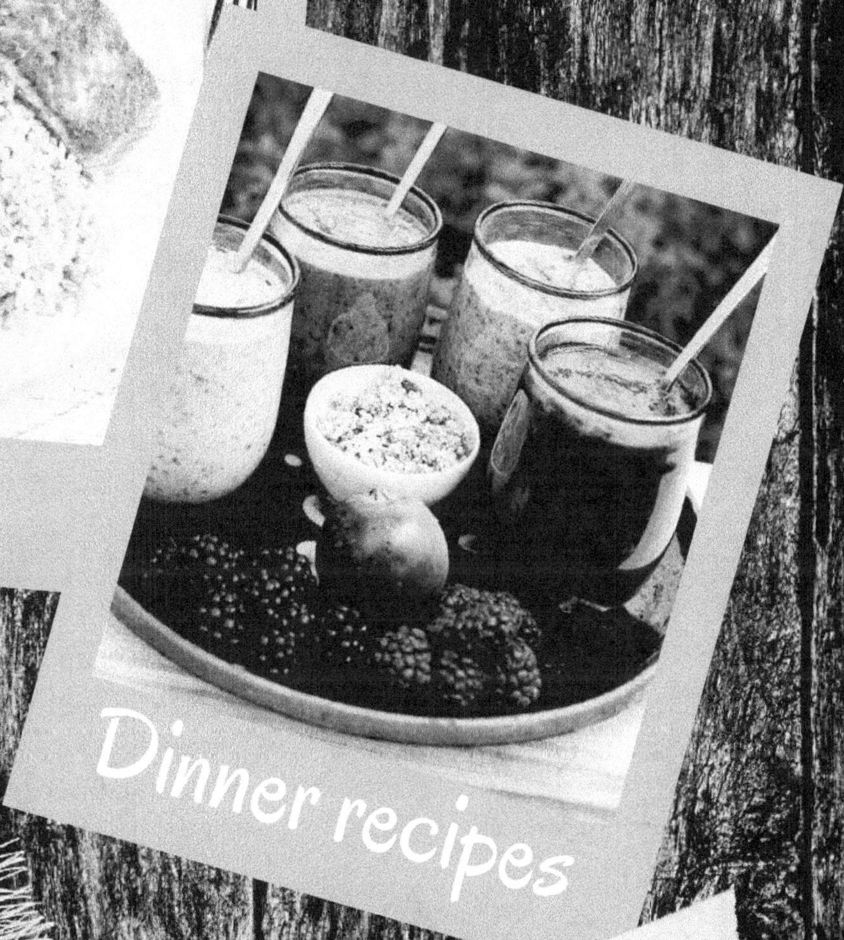

Dinner recipes

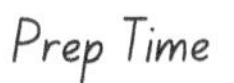

Prep Time

Cook Time

Rating

Difficulty

Instructions

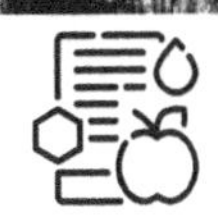

Nutritional Value

Serving

Baked Chicken Breast With Roasted Vegetables

Introduction

Baked chicken breast with roasted vegetables is a nutritious and flavorful option for individuals in Stage 2 of diverticulitis healing and stabilization. This dish features tender and juicy chicken breasts seasoned with herbs and spices, served alongside a colorful assortment of roasted vegetables, providing protein, fiber, vitamins, and minerals to support digestive health and overall well-being.

Ingredients

- 4 boneless, skinless chicken breasts
- 2 cups mixed vegetables (such as carrots, bell peppers, zucchini, and cherry tomatoes), cut into bite-sized pieces
- 2 tablespoons olive oil
- 1 teaspoon garlic powder
- 1 teaspoon onion powder
- 1 teaspoon dried thyme
- 1 teaspoon dried rosemary
- Salt and pepper to taste
- Fresh herbs for garnish (optional)

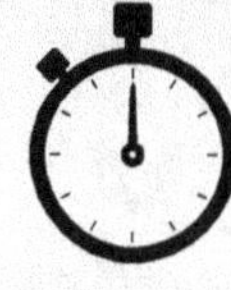  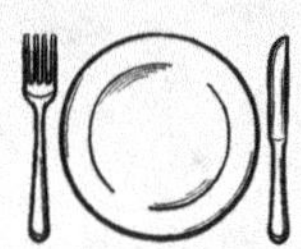

Prep Time 15 mins   **Cook Time** 25-30 mins   **Serving** 4

Preparation Method

1. Preheat the oven to 400°F (200°C).
2. Place the chicken breasts in a baking dish lined with parchment paper.
3. In a small bowl, whisk together the olive oil, garlic powder, onion powder, dried thyme, dried rosemary, salt, and pepper.
4. Brush the olive oil mixture over the chicken breasts, coating them evenly.
5. Arrange the mixed vegetables around the chicken breasts in the baking dish.
6. Drizzle any remaining olive oil mixture over the vegetables.
7. Bake in the preheated oven for 25-30 minutes, or until the chicken is cooked through and the vegetables are tender.
8. Remove from the oven and let rest for a few minutes before serving.
9. Garnish with fresh herbs, if desired.
10. Serve the baked chicken breast with roasted vegetables hot as a wholesome and satisfying meal option.

- Calories: 250 kcal
- Protein: 30g
- Fat: 10g
- Carbohydrates: 10g
- Fiber: 3g
- Sugar: 4g

Difficulty

Rating

2 Turkey Meatballs With Zucchini Noodles

Introduction

Turkey meatballs with zucchini noodles are a light and flavorful option for individuals in Stage 2 of diverticulitis healing and stabilization. This dish features lean turkey meatballs seasoned with herbs and spices, served with fresh zucchini noodles and marinara sauce, providing protein, fiber, vitamins, and minerals to support digestive health and overall well-being.

Ingredients

For the Turkey Meatballs:
- 1 pound ground turkey
- 1/4 cup breadcrumbs (or almond flour for a gluten-free option)
- 1/4 cup grated Parmesan cheese
- 1 egg
- 2 cloves garlic, minced
- 1 teaspoon dried Italian herbs (such as oregano, basil, and parsley)
- Salt and pepper to taste
- 2 tablespoons olive oil

For the Zucchini Noodles:
- 4 medium zucchini, spiralized into noodles
- 1 cup marinara sauce
- Fresh basil leaves for garnish (optional)

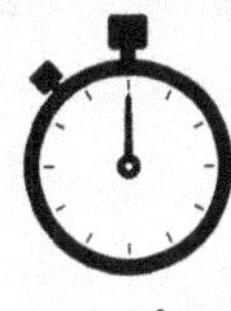

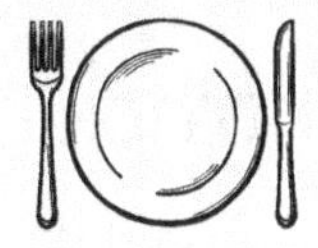

Prep Time	Cook Time	Serving
20 mins	25-30 mins	4

Preparation Method

1. Preheat the oven to 400°F (200°C).
2. In a large mixing bowl, combine the ground turkey, breadcrumbs (or almond flour), grated Parmesan cheese, egg, minced garlic, dried Italian herbs, salt, and pepper. Mix well to combine.
3. Shape the turkey mixture into meatballs, about 1 inch in diameter.
4. The olive oil should be heated up over medium heat, using a large skillet.
5. Add the turkey meatballs to the skillet and cook until browned on all sides, about 5-7 minutes.
6. Transfer the browned meatballs to a baking dish and bake in the preheated oven for 15-20 minutes, or until cooked through.
7. In the same skillet, add the spiralized zucchini noodles and marinara sauce. Cook until the zucchini noodles are tender, about 5 minutes.
8. Remove the turkey meatballs from the oven and let rest for a few minutes.
9. Serve the turkey meatballs over the zucchini noodles, garnished with fresh basil leaves, if desired.
10. Enjoy the turkey meatballs with zucchini noodles hot as a delicious and nutritious meal option.

- Calories: 300 kcal
- Protein: 25g
- Fat: 15g
- Carbohydrates: 15g
- Fiber: 5g
- Sugar: 4g

Difficulty

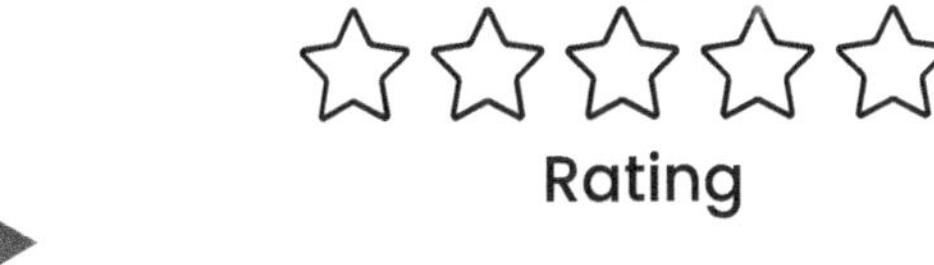

Rating

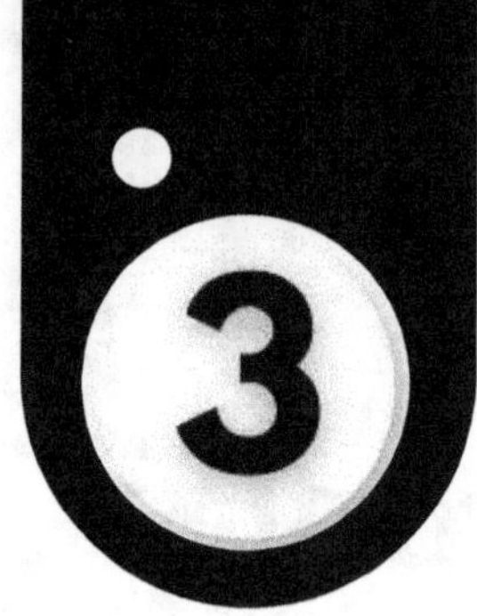

Quinoa-Stuffed Bell Peppers

Introduction

Quinoa-stuffed bell peppers are a nutritious and satisfying option for individuals in Stage 2 of diverticulitis healing and stabilization. This dish features colorful bell peppers stuffed with a flavorful mixture of quinoa, vegetables, and spices, providing protein, fiber, vitamins, and minerals to support digestive health and overall well-being.

Ingredients

- 4 large bell peppers (any color), halved and seeds removed
- 1 cup quinoa, rinsed
- 2 cups vegetable broth
- 1 tablespoon olive oil
- 1 small onion, diced
- 2 cloves garlic, minced
- 1 cup diced tomatoes
- 1 cup cooked black beans
- 1 cup corn kernels
- 1 teaspoon chili powder
- 1 teaspoon ground cumin
- Salt and pepper to taste
- Optional toppings: chopped fresh cilantro, avocado slices, Greek yogurt or sour cream

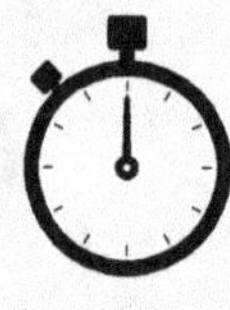
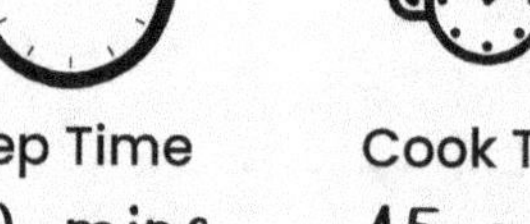

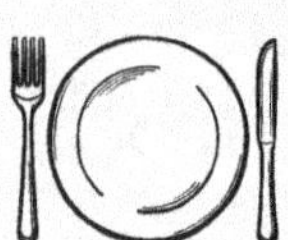

Prep Time 20 mins

Cook Time 45 mins

Serving 4

Preparation Method

1. Preheat the oven to 375°F (190°C).
2. Place the bell pepper halves cut-side up in a baking dish.
3. Mix/combine the quinoa and vegetable broth in a medium sized saucepan. Bring to a boil, then reduce the heat to low, cover, and simmer for 15-20 minutes, or until the quinoa is cooked and the liquid is absorbed.
4. The olive oil should be heated up over medium heat, using a large skillet. Add the chopped garlic and onion, and sauté for about 5 minutes, or until they're soft and tender.
5. Add the diced tomatoes, cooked black beans, corn kernels, chili powder, ground cumin, salt, and pepper to the skillet. Cook for an additional 5 minutes, until heated through.
6. Stir the cooked quinoa into the vegetable mixture until well combined.
7. Spoon the quinoa mixture evenly into the bell pepper halves.
8. Cover the baking dish with aluminum foil and bake in the preheated oven for 25-30 minutes, or until the bell peppers are tender.
9. Take out of the oven and allow it to cool down a little before serving.
10. Garnish with optional toppings such as chopped fresh cilantro, avocado slices, or Greek yogurt/sour cream.
11. Serve the quinoa-stuffed bell peppers hot as a flavorful and nutritious meal option.

- Calories: 300 kcal
- Protein: 10g
- Fat: 6g
- Carbohydrates: 55g
- Fiber: 12g
- Sugar: 8g

Difficulty

Rating

Grilled Chicken Tacos

Introduction

Grilled fish tacos are a delicious and wholesome option for individuals in Stage 2 of diverticulitis healing and stabilization. This dish features tender and flaky grilled fish fillets wrapped in warm corn tortillas and topped with crunchy cabbage slaw, fresh salsa, and creamy avocado, providing protein, fiber, healthy fats, and essential nutrients to support digestive health and overall well-being.

Ingredients

For the Grilled Fish:
- 4 white fish fillets (such as tilapia, cod, or halibut)
- 2 tablespoons olive oil
- 1 teaspoon chili powder
- 1 teaspoon ground cumin
- 1 teaspoon paprika
- Salt and pepper to taste

For the Cabbage Slaw:
- 2 cups shredded cabbage (red or green)
- 1/4 cup chopped fresh cilantro
- 1 tablespoon olive oil
- 1 tablespoon lime juice
- Salt and pepper to taste

For Serving:
- 8 small corn tortillas, warmed
- Fresh salsa
- Sliced avocado
- Lime wedges

Difficulty

 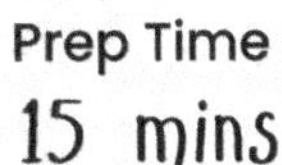  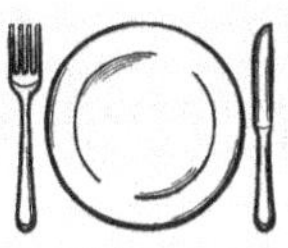

Prep Time	Cook Time	Serving
15 mins	10 mins	4

Preparation Method

1. Your grill or grill pan should be preheated over medium-high heat.
2. In a small bowl, whisk together the olive oil, chili powder, ground cumin, paprika, salt, and pepper.
3. Brush the fish fillets with the olive oil mixture, coating them evenly.
4. Grill the fish fillets for 3-4 minutes per side, or until cooked through and flaky.
5. In a large mixing bowl, combine the shredded cabbage, chopped fresh cilantro, olive oil, lime juice, salt, and pepper. Toss until well coated.
6. To assemble the tacos, place a grilled fish fillet on each warmed corn tortilla.
7. Top with a generous amount of cabbage slaw, fresh salsa, and sliced avocado.
8. Serve the grilled fish tacos with lime wedges on the side for squeezing.
9. Enjoy the grilled fish tacos hot as a flavorful and satisfying meal option.

- Calories: 300 kcal
- Protein: 20g
- Fat: 10g
- Carbohydrates: 30g
- Fiber: 6g
- Sugar: 4g

Rating

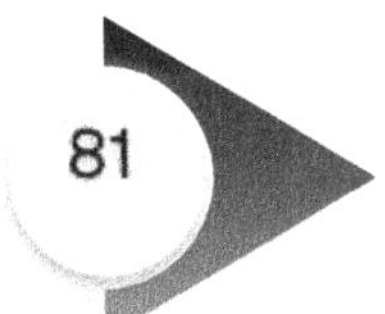

5 Shrimp and Vegetable Stir-Fry

Introduction

Shrimp and vegetable stir-fry is a flavorful and nutrient-rich dish that is perfect for individuals in Stage 2 of diverticulitis healing and stabilization. This dish features succulent shrimp, crisp vegetables, and aromatic spices stir-fried to perfection, providing protein, fiber, vitamins, and minerals to support digestive health and overall well-being.

Ingredients

- 1 pound large shrimp, peeled and deveined
- 2 cups mixed vegetables (such as bell peppers, broccoli, snap peas, carrots, and mushrooms), sliced
- 2 cloves garlic, minced
- 1-inch piece of ginger, grated
- 2 tablespoons low-sodium soy sauce (or tamari for a gluten-free option)
- 1 tablespoon rice vinegar
- 1 tablespoon honey (or maple syrup for a vegan option)
- 1 tablespoon sesame oil
- 2 tablespoons vegetable oil
- Cooked brown rice or quinoa, for serving
- Optional garnishes: sliced green onions, sesame seeds, cilantro

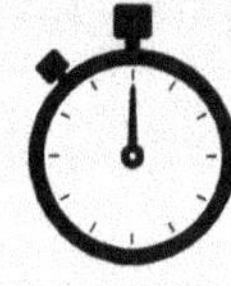
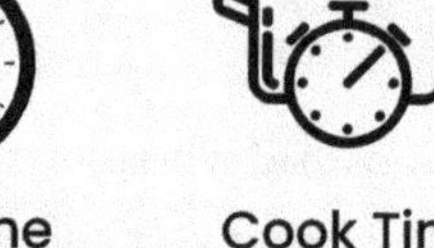
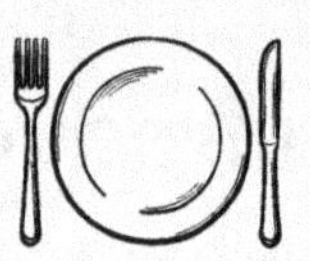

Prep Time 15 mins   **Cook Time** 10 mins   **Serving** 4

Preparation Method

1. In a small bowl, whisk together the minced garlic, grated ginger, low-sodium soy sauce, rice vinegar, honey, and sesame oil to make the sauce. Set aside.
2. Heat one tablespoon of vegetable oil in a large skillet or wok over medium-high heat.
3. Add the shrimp to the skillet and stir-fry for 2-3 minutes, or until pink and opaque. Take the shrimp out of the skillet and set aside.
4. Add the remaining tablespoon of vegetable oil to the skillet.
5. Add the mixed vegetables to the skillet and stir-fry for 3-4 minutes, or until crisp-tender.
6. Return the cooked shrimp to the skillet.
7. Pour the sauce over the shrimp and vegetables in the skillet. Stir well to combine and coat everything evenly with the sauce.
8. Continue to cook for an additional 1-2 minutes, or until the sauce has thickened slightly.
9. Remove from heat and serve the shrimp and vegetable stir-fry hot over cooked brown rice or quinoa.
10. Garnish with sliced green onions, sesame seeds, and cilantro, if desired.
11. Enjoy the shrimp and vegetable stir-fry as a delicious and nutritious meal option.

- Calories: 250 kcal
- Protein: 20g
- Fat: 10g
- Carbohydrates: 20g
- Fiber: 4g
- Sugar: 8g

Difficulty

Rating

Lentil and Vegetable Curry

Introduction

Lentil and vegetable curry is a comforting and nourishing dish that is ideal for individuals in Stage 2 of diverticulitis healing and stabilization. This dish features hearty lentils, vibrant vegetables, and aromatic spices simmered in a rich and flavorful curry sauce, providing protein, fiber, vitamins, and minerals to support digestive health and overall well-being.

Ingredients

- 1 cup dried green or brown lentils, rinsed
- 3 cups vegetable broth
- 1 tablespoon olive oil
- 1 onion, diced
- 2 cloves garlic, minced
- 1-inch piece of ginger, grated
- 2 carrots, diced
- 1 bell pepper, diced
- 1 zucchini, diced
- 1 can (14 oz) diced tomatoes
- 1 can (14 oz) coconut milk
- 2 tablespoons curry powder
- 1 teaspoon ground cumin
- 1 teaspoon ground turmeric
- Salt and pepper to taste
- Cooked brown rice or quinoa, for serving
- Fresh cilantro, for garnish

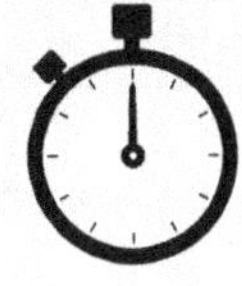

Prep Time
15 mins

Cook Time
45 mins

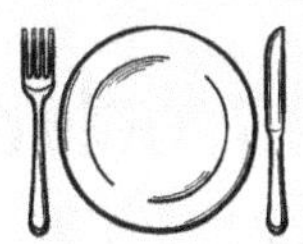

Serving
4

Preparation Method

1. In a large pot, combine the dried lentils and vegetable broth. Bring to a boil, then reduce the heat to low, cover, and simmer for 20-25 minutes, or until the lentils are tender.
2. While the lentils are cooking, heat the olive oil in a large skillet over medium heat.
3. Add the diced onion to the skillet and sauté until softened, about 5 minutes.
4. Stir in the minced garlic and grated ginger, and cook for an additional 1-2 minutes, until fragrant.
5. Add the diced carrots, bell pepper, and zucchini to the skillet. Cook for about 5-7 minutes, or until the vegetables are soft and tender.
6. Stir in the diced tomatoes (with their juices), coconut milk, curry powder, ground cumin, ground turmeric, salt, and pepper. Bring to a simmer and cook for 10-15 minutes, allowing the flavors to meld together.
7. Once the lentils are tender, add them to the skillet with the vegetable curry mixture. Stir well to combine.
8. Continue to simmer for an additional 5-10 minutes, until heated through.
9. Taste and adjust the seasoning, if necessary.
10. Serve the lentil and vegetable curry hot over cooked brown rice or quinoa.
11. Garnish with fresh cilantro before serving.
12. Enjoy the lentil and vegetable curry as a hearty and satisfying meal option.

- Calories: 350 kcal
- Protein: 15g
- Fat: 15g
- Carbohydrates: 40g
- Fiber: 12g
- Sugar: 8g

Difficulty

Rating

Turkey and Bean Chili

Introduction

Turkey and bean chili is a comforting and nutritious dish that is perfect for individuals in Stage 2 of diverticulitis healing and stabilization. This flavorful chili features lean ground turkey, hearty beans, and aromatic spices simmered to perfection, providing protein, fiber, vitamins, and minerals to support digestive health and overall well-being.

Ingredients

- 1 pound lean ground turkey
- 1 tablespoon olive oil
- 1 onion, diced
- 2 cloves garlic, minced
- 1 bell pepper, diced
- 1 jalapeno pepper, seeded and diced (optional)
- 1 can (14 oz) diced tomatoes
- 1 can (14 oz) kidney beans, drained and rinsed
- 1 can (14 oz) black beans, drained and rinsed
- 2 cups low-sodium vegetable broth
- 2 tablespoons chili powder
- 1 teaspoon ground cumin
- 1 teaspoon smoked paprika
- Salt and pepper to taste
- Optional toppings: chopped fresh cilantro, sliced green onions, shredded cheese, Greek yogurt or sour cream

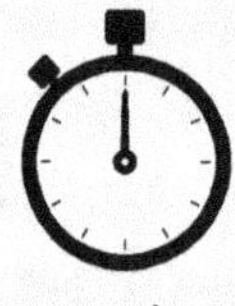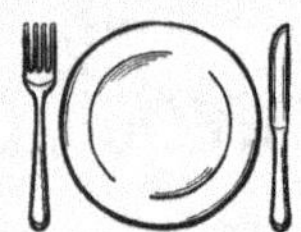

Prep Time	Cook Time	Serving
15 mins	40 mins	6

Preparation Method

1. The olive oil should be heated up over medium heat, using a large pot or Dutch oven.
2. Add the diced onion, minced garlic, diced bell pepper, and diced jalapeno pepper (if using) to the pot. Sauté the vegetables for about five to seven minutes, or until they are soft and tender.
3. Add the ground turkey to the pot and cook, breaking it up with a spoon, until browned and cooked through, about 5-7 minutes.
4. Stir in the diced tomatoes, kidney beans, black beans, vegetable broth, chili powder, ground cumin, smoked paprika, salt, and pepper.
5. Bring the chili to a simmer, then turn the heat down to low. Cover and simmer for 20-25 minutes, stirring occasionally, to allow the flavors to meld together.
6. Taste and adjust the seasoning, if necessary.
7. Serve the turkey and bean chili hot, garnished with optional toppings such as chopped fresh cilantro, sliced green onions, shredded cheese, or Greek yogurt/sour cream.
8. Enjoy the turkey and bean chili as a hearty and satisfying meal option.

- Calories: 300 kcal
- Protein: 25g
- Fat: 10g
- Carbohydrates: 25g
- Fiber: 8g
- Sugar: 5g

Difficulty

Rating

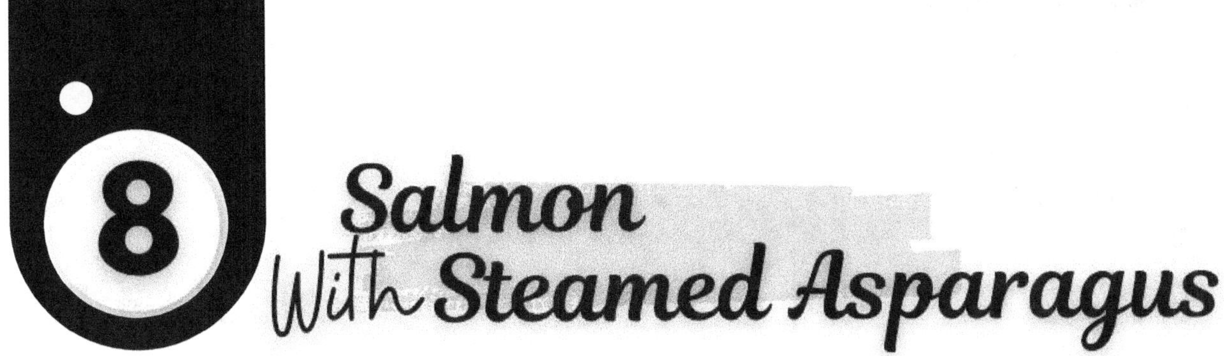

Introduction

Salmon with steamed asparagus is a nutritious and flavorful dish that is perfect for individuals in Stage 2 of diverticulitis healing and stabilization. This dish features tender and flaky salmon fillets paired with vibrant asparagus spears, providing omega-3 fatty acids, vitamins, and minerals to support digestive health and overall well-being.

Ingredients

- 4 salmon fillets
- 1 tablespoon olive oil
- Salt and pepper to taste
- 1 bunch asparagus, tough ends trimmed
- Lemon wedges, for serving
- Optional garnishes: chopped fresh parsley, lemon zest

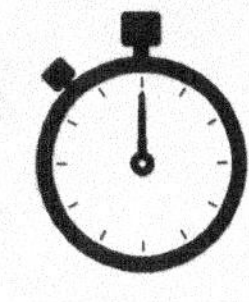 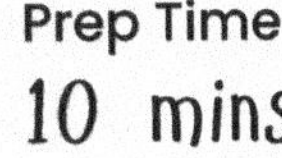  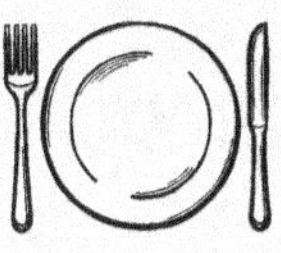

Prep Time 10 mins **Cook Time** 15 mins **Serving** 4

Preparation Method

1. Preheat the oven to 400°F (200°C).
2. Place the salmon fillets on a baking sheet lined with parchment paper.
3. Drizzle the salmon fillets with olive oil and season with salt and pepper.
4. Roast in the preheated oven for 12-15 minutes, or until the salmon is cooked through and flakes easily with a fork.
5. While the salmon is cooking, steam the asparagus spears until tender, about 5-7 minutes.
6. To serve, divide the steamed asparagus among plates and top with the roasted salmon fillets.
7. Squeeze fresh lemon juice over the salmon and asparagus, and garnish with optional chopped fresh parsley and lemon zest.
8. Enjoy the salmon with steamed asparagus as a delicious and nutritious meal option.

Calories: 250 kcal
- Protein: 25g
- Fat: 15g
- Carbohydrates: 5g
- Fiber: 3g
- Sugar: 2g

Difficulty

Rating

Chicken and Vegetable Skewers

Introduction

Chicken and vegetable skewers are a delicious and nutritious dish that is perfect for individuals in Stage 2 of diverticulitis healing and stabilization. These skewers feature tender pieces of chicken breast and colorful vegetables, seasoned with aromatic herbs and spices, providing protein, fiber, vitamins, and minerals to support digestive health and overall well-being.

Ingredients

- 1 pound boneless, skinless chicken breast, cut into bite-sized pieces
- 1 red bell pepper, cut into chunks
- 1 yellow bell pepper, cut into chunks
- 1 red onion, cut into chunks
- 1 zucchini, sliced into rounds
- 8-10 cherry tomatoes
- 2 tablespoons olive oil
- 2 cloves garlic, minced
- 1 teaspoon dried oregano
- 1 teaspoon dried thyme
- 1 teaspoon paprika
- Salt and pepper to taste
- Wooden skewers, soaked in water for 30 minutes

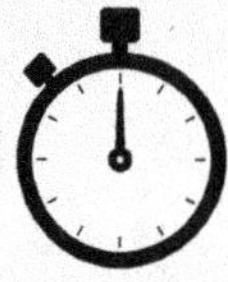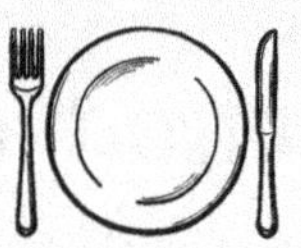

Prep Time	Cook Time	Serving
15 mins	10-12 mins	4

Preparation Method

1. Preheat the grill to medium-high heat.
2. In a large bowl, combine the chicken breast pieces, bell pepper chunks, onion chunks, zucchini slices, and cherry tomatoes.
3. In a small bowl, whisk together the olive oil, minced garlic, dried oregano, dried thyme, paprika, salt, and pepper.
4. Pour the olive oil mixture over the chicken and vegetables in the large bowl. Toss well to coat everything evenly.
5. Thread the marinated chicken and vegetables onto the soaked wooden skewers, alternating between chicken and vegetables.
6. Place the skewers on the preheated grill and cook for 10-12 minutes, turning occasionally, until the chicken is cooked through and the vegetables are tender and slightly charred.
7. The skewers should be taken off the grill and placed on a serving plate.
8. Serve the chicken and vegetable skewers hot, accompanied by cooked quinoa, rice, or a side salad, if desired.
9. Enjoy the chicken and vegetable skewers as a flavorful and nutritious meal option.

- Calories: 250 kcal
- Protein: 25g
- Fat: 10g
- Carbohydrates: 15g
- Fiber: 4g
- Sugar: 6g

Difficulty

Rating

Veggie and Quinoa Stuffed Portobello Mushrooms

Introduction

Veggie and quinoa stuffed portobello mushrooms are a satisfying and nutrient-rich dish that is perfect for individuals in Stage 2 of diverticulitis healing and stabilization. These hearty mushrooms are filled with a flavorful mixture of cooked quinoa, sautéed vegetables, and savory herbs, providing protein, fiber, vitamins, and minerals to support digestive health and overall well-being.

Ingredients

- 4 large portobello mushrooms, stems removed
- 1 cup cooked quinoa
- 1 tablespoon olive oil
- 1 onion, diced
- 2 cloves garlic, minced
- 1 bell pepper, diced
- 1 zucchini, diced
- 1 cup baby spinach, chopped
- 1 teaspoon dried Italian herbs (such as basil, oregano, and thyme)
- Salt and pepper to taste
- ½ cup grated Parmesan cheese (optional)
- Fresh parsley, for garnish

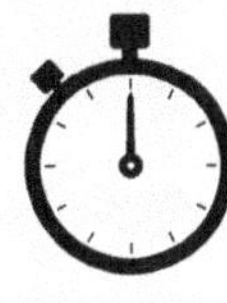

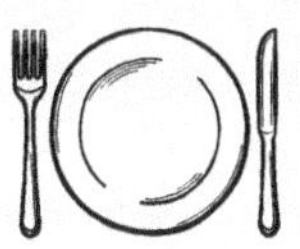

Prep Time	Cook Time	Serving
20 mins	20-25 mins	4

Preparation Method

1. Preheat the oven to 375°F (190°C).
2. Place the portobello mushrooms on a baking sheet lined with parchment paper, gill side up.
3. The olive oil should be heated up over medium heat, using a large skillet.
4. Add the diced onion and minced garlic to the skillet. Saute for about 5 minutes, or until tender and aromatic.
5. Add the diced bell pepper and diced zucchini to the skillet. Simmer for a further five to seven minutes, or until the veggies are soft and tender.
6. Stir in the chopped baby spinach and dried Italian herbs. Cook for about 2-3 minutes, or until the spinach has wilted.
7. Remove the skillet from heat and stir in the cooked quinoa. Season with salt and pepper to taste.
8. Spoon the quinoa and vegetable mixture into the cavity of each portobello mushroom, dividing evenly among the mushrooms.
9. If using, sprinkle the grated Parmesan cheese over the stuffed mushrooms.
10. Bake in the preheated oven for 20-25 minutes, or until the mushrooms are tender and the filling is heated through.
11. Remove from the oven and garnish with fresh parsley before serving.
12. Enjoy the veggie and quinoa stuffed portobello mushrooms as a delicious and nutritious meal option.

- Calories: 200 kcal
- Protein: 8g
- Fat: 5g
- Carbohydrates: 30g
- Fiber: 6g
- Sugar: 4g

Difficulty

Rating

STAGE 3: MAINTENANCE AND PREVENTION RECIPE

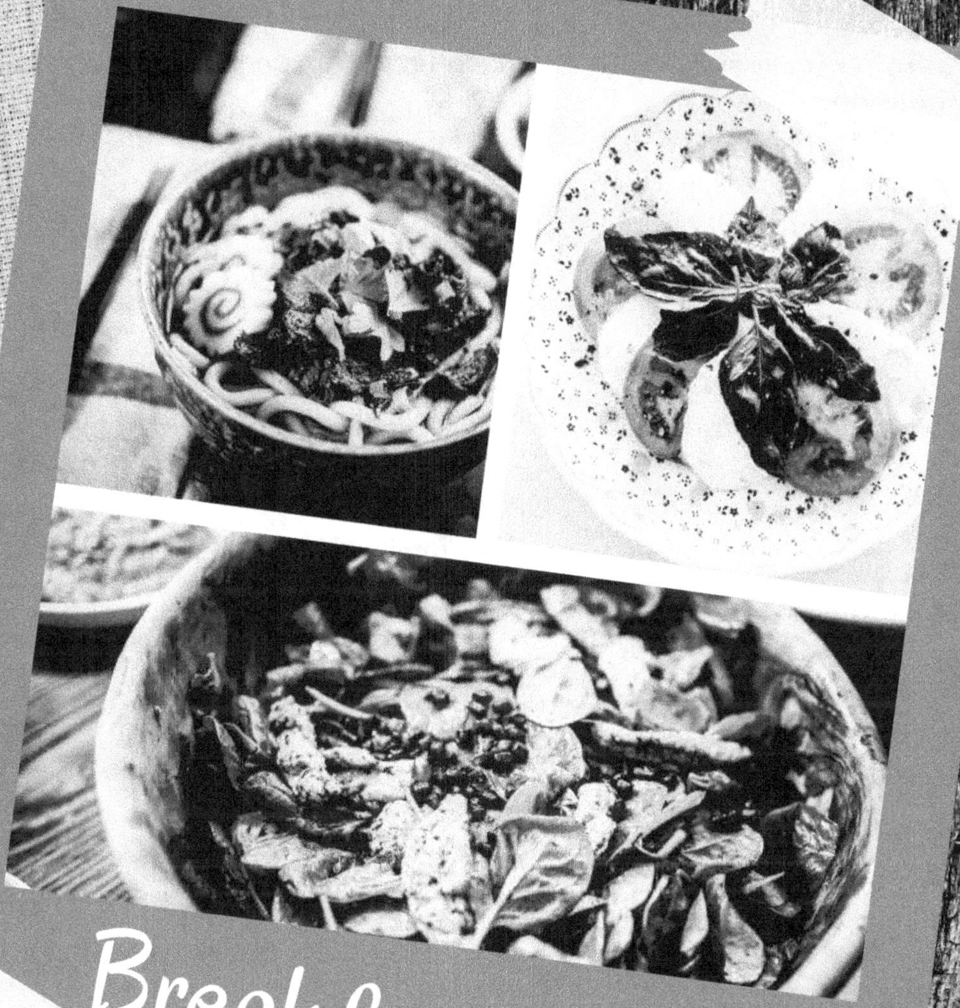

Breakfast recipes

Prep Time

Cook Time

Rating

Difficulty

Instructions

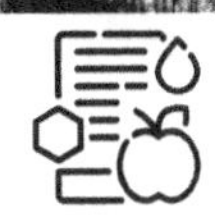

Nutritional Value

Serving

Chia Seed Breakfast Bowl

Introduction

A chia seed breakfast bowl is a nutritious and satisfying dish that is perfect for individuals in Stage 3 of diverticulitis maintenance and prevention. This breakfast bowl features chia seeds soaked in almond milk and topped with fresh fruits, nuts, and seeds, providing a rich source of fiber, omega-3 fatty acids, vitamins, and minerals to support digestive health and overall well-being.

Ingredients

- 1/4 cup chia seeds
- 1 cup unsweetened almond milk
- 1/2 teaspoon vanilla extract
- 1 tablespoon honey or maple syrup (optional)
- Assorted fresh fruits (such as berries, sliced banana, and diced mango)
- Nuts and seeds (such as chopped almonds, pumpkin seeds, and shredded coconut)
- Additional toppings (such as Greek yogurt, granola, or nut butter)

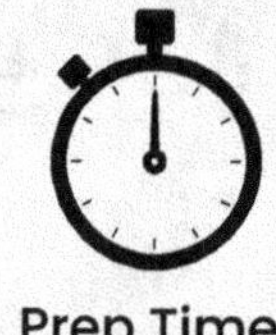

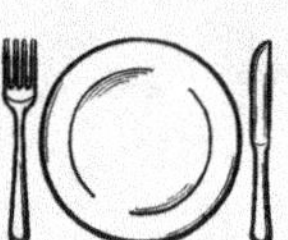

Prep Time
5 mins
(Plus Chilling Time)

Cook Time
0 mins

Serving
2

Preparation Method

1. In a small bowl or mason jar, combine the chia seeds, almond milk, vanilla extract, and honey or maple syrup (if using). Stir well to combine.
2. Cover the bowl or jar and refrigerate for at least 2 hours, preferably overnight, to allow the chia seeds to absorb the liquid and thicken into a pudding-like consistency.
3. Once the chia seed pudding has set, give it a good stir to break up any clumps.
4. Transfer the chia seed pudding to serving bowls.
5. Top the chia seed pudding with assorted fresh fruits, nuts, seeds, and any additional toppings of your choice.
6. Serve the chia seed breakfast bowls immediately and enjoy a delicious and nutritious start to your day.

- Calories: 180 kcal
- Protein: 5g
- Fat: 9g
- Carbohydrates: 20g
- Fiber: 10g
- Sugar: 5g

Difficulty

Rating

2 Sweet Potato Hash with Poached Eggs

Introduction

Sweet potato hash with poached eggs is a flavorful and nutritious dish that is perfect for individuals in Stage 3 of diverticulitis maintenance and prevention. This hearty hash features diced sweet potatoes, bell peppers, onions, and savory spices, topped with perfectly poached eggs, providing a rich source of fiber, vitamins, and minerals to support digestive health and overall well-being.

Ingredients

- 2 medium sweet potatoes, peeled and diced
- 1 tablespoon olive oil
- 1 bell pepper, diced
- 1 onion, diced
- 2 cloves garlic, minced
- 1 teaspoon smoked paprika
- 1/2 teaspoon ground cumin
- Salt and pepper to taste
- 4 large eggs
- Fresh parsley, chopped, for garnish (optional)

 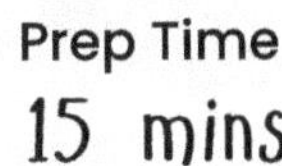  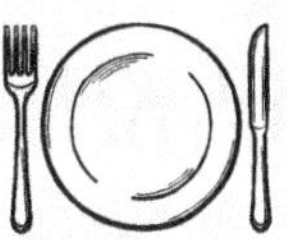

Prep Time 15 mins

Cook Time 20 mins

Serving 2

Preparation Method

1. The olive oil should be heated up over medium heat, using a large skillet.

2. Add the diced sweet potatoes to the skillet and cook, stirring occasionally, for 5-7 minutes, or until they begin to soften.

3. Add the diced bell pepper, diced onion, minced garlic, smoked paprika, ground cumin, salt, and pepper to the skillet. Stir well to combine.

4. Continue to cook the sweet potato hash, stirring occasionally, for an additional 8-10 minutes, or until the sweet potatoes are tender and lightly browned.

5. While the sweet potato hash is cooking, prepare the poached eggs. Pour water into a big saucepan and heat it gently over medium heat to bring it to a moderate simmer. Each egg should be cracked into a ramekin or small bowl.

6. Using a slotted spoon, carefully lower each egg into the simmering water and cook for 3-4 minutes, or until the whites are set but the yolks are still runny.

7. Use the slotted spoon to remove the poached eggs from the water and drain them on a clean kitchen towel.

8. Divide the sweet potato hash among serving plates and top each portion with a poached egg.

9. If preferred you can garnish with chopped fresh parsley.

10. Serve the sweet potato hash with poached eggs hot and enjoy a delicious and satisfying meal.

- Calories: 300 kcal
- Protein: 10g
- Fat: 12g
- Carbohydrates: 40g
- Fiber: 8g
- Sugar: 10g

Difficulty

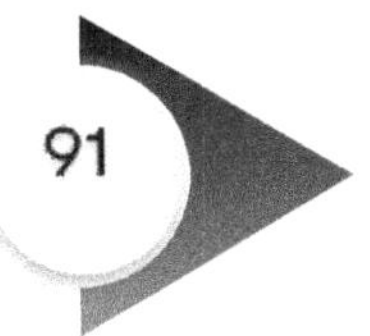

Rating

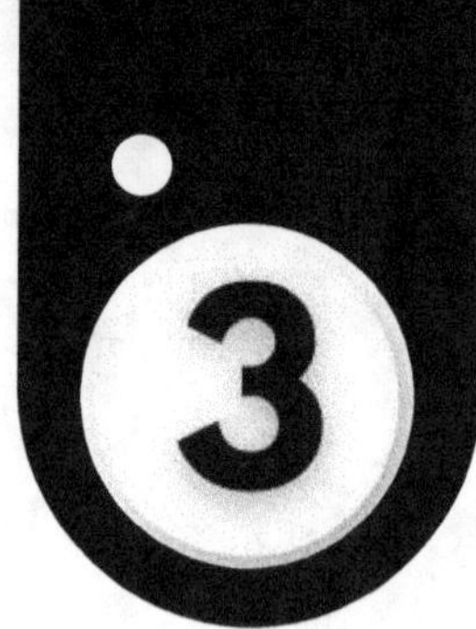

3 Buckwheat Pancakes with Blueberry Compote

Introduction

Buckwheat pancakes with blueberry compote are a delightful and nutritious option for individuals in Stage 3 of diverticulitis maintenance and prevention. These fluffy pancakes are made with wholesome buckwheat flour and topped with a sweet and tangy blueberry compote, providing fiber, antioxidants, vitamins, and minerals to support digestive health and overall well-being.

Ingredients

Ingredients for Buckwheat Pancakes:
- 1 cup buckwheat flour
- 1 tablespoon baking powder
- 1 tablespoon sugar (optional)
- 1/4 teaspoon salt
- 1 cup milk (dairy or plant-based)
- 1 large egg
- 2 tablespoons melted butter or oil
- Butter or oil for cooking

Ingredients for Blueberry Compote:
- 1 cup fresh or frozen blueberries
- 2 tablespoons water
- 1 tablespoon honey or maple syrup
- 1 teaspoon lemon juice
- 1/2 teaspoon vanilla extract

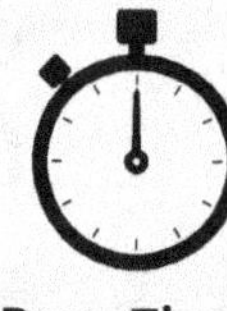  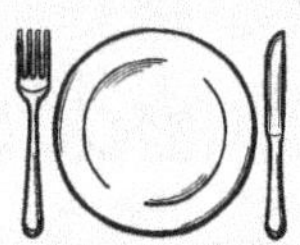

Prep Time	Cook Time	Serving
10 mins	15 mins	4

Preparation Method

Preparation Method for Buckwheat Pancakes:
1. In a large mixing bowl, whisk together the buckwheat flour, baking powder, sugar (if using), and salt.
2. Beat/whisk the egg, milk, and melted butter or oil in another bowl.
3. Add and pour-in the wet ingredients into the dry ingredients and stir until they're well blended/combined. Be careful not to overmix; a few lumps are okay.
4. Heat a non-stick skillet or griddle over medium heat and lightly grease with butter or oil.
5. For each pancake, pour 1/4 cup of batter to the skillet. Fry until bubbles develop on the surface, then turn and cook until both sides of the pancake are golden brown.
6. Repeat with the remaining batter, adjusting the heat as needed to prevent burning.

Preparation Method for Blueberry Compote:
1. In a small saucepan, combine the blueberries, water, honey or maple syrup, lemon juice, and vanilla extract.
2. Bring the mixture to a simmer over medium heat, then reduce the heat to low and cook for 5-7 minutes, stirring occasionally, until the blueberries have softened and released their juices.
3. Remove from heat and allow it cool slightly before serving.

- Calories: 200 kcal
- Protein: 6g
- Fat: 7g
- Carbohydrates: 30g
- Fiber: 4g
- Sugar: 4g

Difficulty

Rating

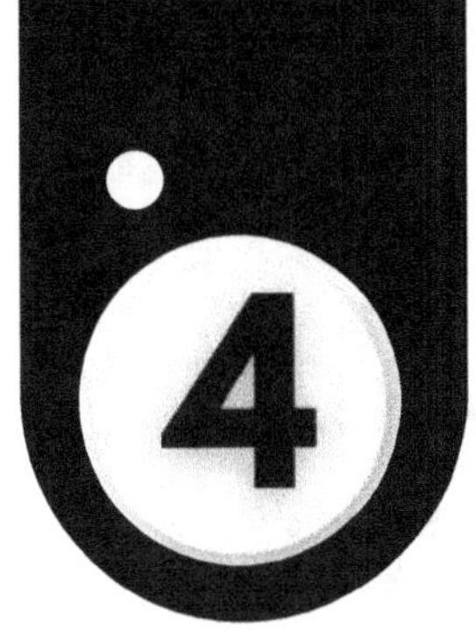

Veggie Omelette

Introduction

A veggie omelette is a delicious and nutritious dish that is perfect for individuals in Stage 3 of diverticulitis maintenance and prevention. This fluffy omelette is filled with a colorful assortment of sautéed vegetables and savory herbs, providing fiber, vitamins, minerals, and protein to support digestive health and overall well-being.

Ingredients

- 4 large eggs
- 2 tablespoons milk (dairy or plant-based)
- Salt and pepper to taste
- 1 tablespoon olive oil
- 1/2 bell pepper, diced
- 1/2 onion, diced
- 1/2 cup sliced mushrooms
- 1/2 cup baby spinach leaves
- 1/4 cup grated cheese (optional)
- Fresh herbs (such as parsley or chives), for garnish

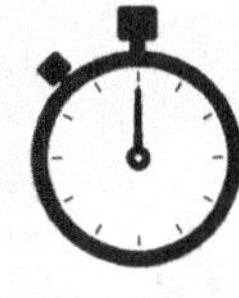
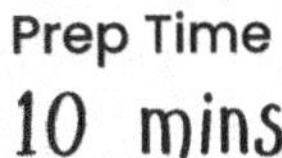

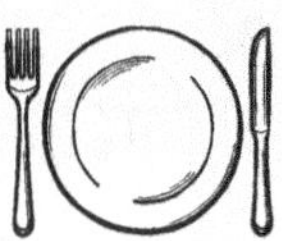

Prep Time 10 mins   **Cook Time** 10 mins   **Serving** 1

Preparation Method

1. Crack the eggs into a bowl, add the milk, salt, and pepper, and whisk until well combined.

2. Heat the olive oil in a non-stick skillet over medium heat.

3. Add the diced bell pepper and onion to the skillet and cook until softened, about 3-4 minutes.

4. Add the sliced mushrooms to the skillet and cook for an additional 2-3 minutes, until they begin to brown.

5. Add the baby spinach leaves to the skillet and cook until wilted, about 1 minute.

6. Pour the beaten eggs over the vegetables in the skillet, tilting the pan to spread them evenly.

7. Cook the omelette for 2-3 minutes, or until the edges start to set.

8. If using, sprinkle the grated cheese over one half of the omelette.

9. Using a spatula, fold the other half of the omelette over the cheese and cook for another minute, until the cheese is melted and the eggs are fully cooked.

10. Slide the veggie omelette onto a plate, garnish with fresh herbs, and serve hot.

- Calories: 300 kcal
- Protein: 20g
- Fat: 20g
- Carbohydrates: 10g
- Fiber: 3g

Difficulty

Rating

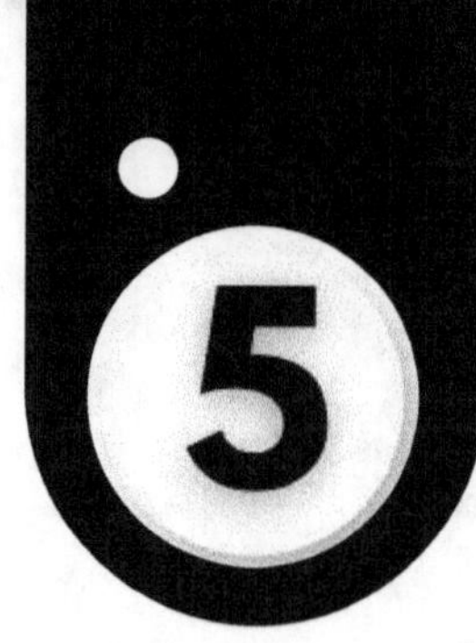

5 Greek Yogurt Parfait With Almond Granola

Introduction

Start your day on a nutritious note with this delicious Greek yogurt parfait topped with crunchy almond granola. Packed with protein, fiber, and healthy fats, this parfait is perfect for individuals in Stage 3 of diverticulitis maintenance and prevention. It's a satisfying and wholesome breakfast option that will keep you energized throughout the morning.

Ingredients

- 1 cup Greek yogurt
- 1/2 cup almond granola
- 1/2 cup mixed berries (such as strawberries, blueberries, and raspberries)
- 1 tablespoon honey or maple syrup (optional)
- Fresh mint leaves, for garnish

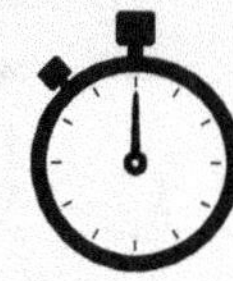 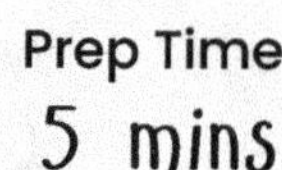  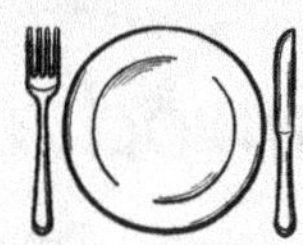

Prep Time
5 mins

Cook Time
0 mins

Serving
1

Preparation Method

1. Spoon half of the Greek yogurt into a serving glass or bowl.
2. Sprinkle half of the almond granola over the yogurt.
3. Place half of the mixed berries on top of the granola.
4. Drizzle with honey or maple syrup if desired.
5. Repeat the layers with the remaining yogurt, granola, and berries.
6. Garnish with fresh mint leaves.
7. Serve immediately and enjoy!

- Calories: 350 kcal
- Protein: 20g
- Fat: 15g
- Carbohydrates: 40g
- Fiber: 6g
- Sugar: 20g

Difficulty

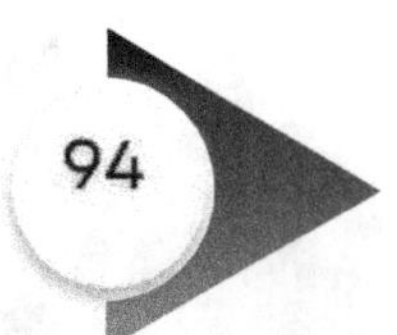

Rating

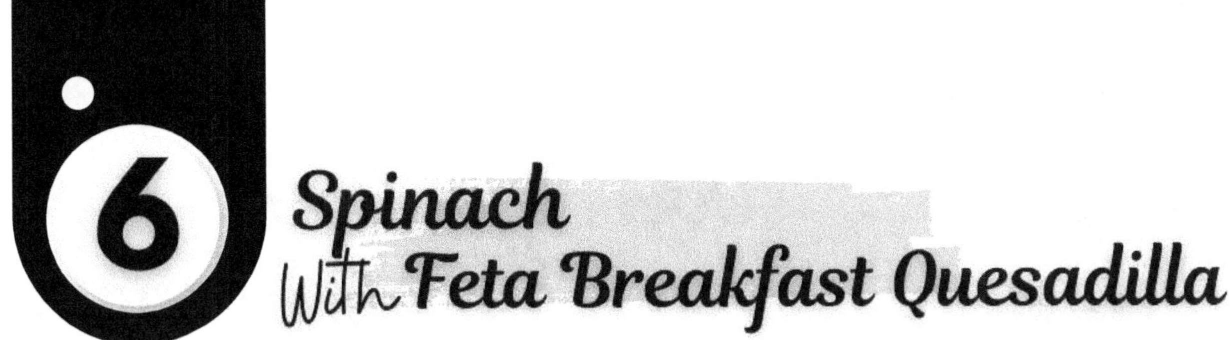

Introduction

This spinach and feta breakfast quesadilla is a flavorful and satisfying option for individuals in Stage 3 of diverticulitis maintenance and prevention. Packed with nutritious ingredients like spinach, feta cheese, and whole grain tortillas, this quesadilla provides fiber, vitamins, minerals, and protein to support digestive health and overall well-being. It's quick and easy to make, making it perfect for busy mornings.

Ingredients

- 2 whole grain tortillas
- 1 cup baby spinach leaves
- 1/4 cup crumbled feta cheese
- 2 large eggs, beaten
- Salt and pepper to taste
- 1 teaspoon olive oil

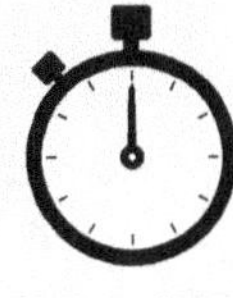
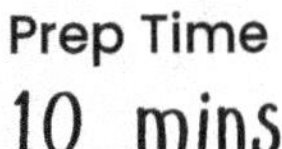

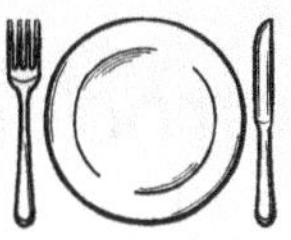

Prep Time	Cook Time	Serving
10 mins	10 mins	1

Preparation Method

1. Heat the olive oil in a non-stick skillet over medium heat.
2. Add the beaten eggs to the skillet and season with salt and pepper.
3. Cook the eggs, stirring occasionally, until they are scrambled and fully cooked.
4. Remove the scrambled eggs from the skillet and set aside.
5. Place one tortilla in the skillet and sprinkle half of the spinach leaves evenly over the tortilla.
6. Spread half of the scrambled eggs and half of the crumbled feta cheese over the spinach.
7. Top with the second tortilla and press down gently.
8. Cook the quesadilla for 2-3 minutes on each side, until golden brown and crispy.
9. Remove from the skillet and let cool slightly before slicing into wedges.
10. Serve warm and enjoy!

- Calories: 400 kcal
- Protein: 25g
- Fat: 20g
- Carbohydrates: 30g
- Fiber: 6g
- Sugar: 2g

Difficulty

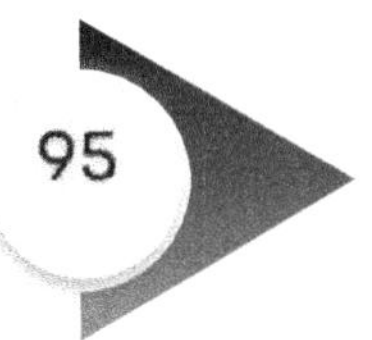

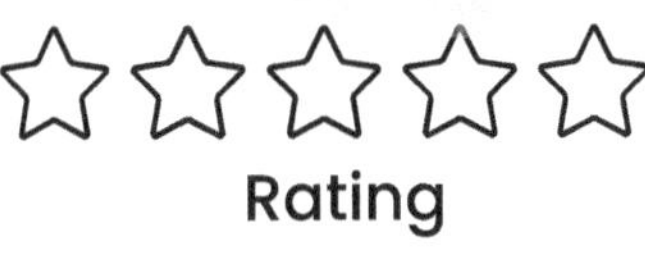

Rating

Overnight Oats
With Peanut Butter and Banana

Introduction

Start your morning off right with these delicious overnight oats with peanut butter and banana. This nutritious and convenient breakfast option is perfect for individuals in Stage 3 of diverticulitis maintenance and prevention. With the creamy texture of oats, the richness of peanut butter, and the sweetness of banana, this recipe is sure to become a favorite.

Ingredients

- 1/2 cup rolled oats
- 1/2 cup milk (dairy or plant-based)
- 1 tablespoon peanut butter
- 1/2 banana, sliced
- 1 teaspoon honey or maple syrup (optional)
- 1 tablespoon chopped nuts or seeds (such as almonds, walnuts, or chia seeds)
- Pinch of cinnamon (optional)

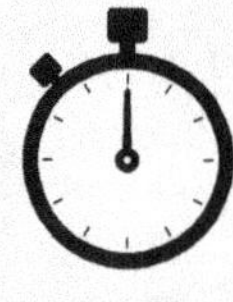  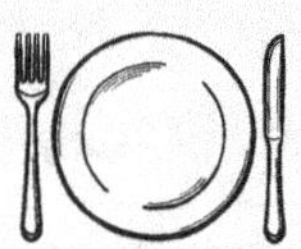

Prep Time	Cook Time	Serving
5 mins	0 mins	1

(Overnight Refrigeration)

Preparation Method

1. In a mason jar or airtight container, combine the rolled oats and milk.
2. Stir in the peanut butter until well incorporated.
3. Add the sliced banana on top of the oat mixture.
4. Drizzle with honey or maple syrup if desired.
5. Sprinkle with chopped nuts or seeds and a pinch of cinnamon.
6. Store the jar or container in the refrigerator for at least 4 hours, or overnight. Make sure to cover it.
7. In the morning, give the oats a good stir before enjoying cold or warmed up in the microwave.
8. Serve and enjoy!

- Calories: 350 kcal
- Protein: 10g
- Fat: 15g
- Carbohydrates: 45g
- Fiber: 7g
- Sugar: 10g

Difficulty

Rating

Smoked Salmon Breakfast Bagel

Introduction

ndulge in a gourmet breakfast with this delicious smoked salmon breakfast bagel. Packed with protein, omega-3 fatty acids, and essential nutrients, this recipe is perfect for individuals in Stage 3 of diverticulitis maintenance and prevention. With the savory flavor of smoked salmon, the creaminess of cream cheese, and the freshness of veggies, this bagel is sure to satisfy your taste buds.

Ingredients

- 1 whole grain or multigrain bagel, sliced and toasted
- 2 tablespoons cream cheese
- 2 slices smoked salmon
- 2 slices tomato
- 2 slices cucumber
- 1 tablespoon chopped red onion
- Fresh dill or chives, for garnish
- Lemon wedges, for serving

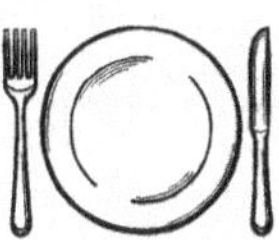

Prep Time
5 mins

Cook Time
5 mins

Serving
1

Preparation Method

1. Spread the cream cheese evenly on each half of the toasted bagel.
2. Layer the smoked salmon slices on the bottom half of the bagel.
3. Top with tomato slices, cucumber slices, and chopped red onion.
4. Garnish with fresh dill or chives.
5. Squeeze lemon juice over the toppings if desired.
6. Place the top half of the bagel over the toppings to form a sandwich.
7. Serve immediately and enjoy!

- Calories: 350 kcal
- Protein: 20g
- Fat: 15g
- Carbohydrates: 30g
- Fiber: 5g
- Sugar: 5g

Difficulty

Rating

Quinoa Breakfast Porridge

Introduction

Start your day with a nutritious and hearty quinoa breakfast porridge. This recipe is perfect for individuals in Stage 3 of diverticulitis maintenance and prevention, providing essential nutrients to support digestive health and overall well-being. Packed with protein, fiber, and vitamins, this porridge will keep you feeling satisfied and energized throughout the morning.

Ingredients

- 1/2 cup quinoa
- 1 cup milk (dairy or plant-based)
- 1/2 teaspoon ground cinnamon
- 1 tablespoon honey or maple syrup (optional)
- 1/4 cup chopped nuts or seeds (such as almonds, walnuts, or pumpkin seeds)
- Fresh berries or sliced fruit, for topping

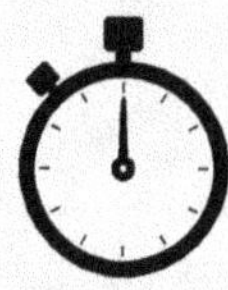  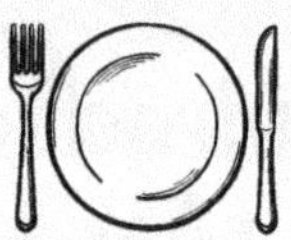

Prep Time 5 mins

Cook Time 20 mins

Serving 2

Preparation Method

1. Rinse the quinoa under cold water in a fine-mesh sieve.
2. In a saucepan, combine the quinoa, milk, and ground cinnamon.
3. Bring the mixture to a boil over medium heat, then reduce the heat to low and simmer for 15-20 minutes, or until the quinoa is tender and the liquid is absorbed.
4. Stir in honey or maple syrup if desired.
5. Remove the saucepan from the heat and let the porridge cool slightly.
6. Divide the porridge into serving bowls and top with chopped nuts or seeds and fresh berries or sliced fruit.
7. Serve warm and enjoy!

- Calories: 300 kcal
- Protein: 10g
- Fat: 10g
- Carbohydrates: 45g
- Fiber: 5g
- Sugar: 10g

Difficulty

Rating

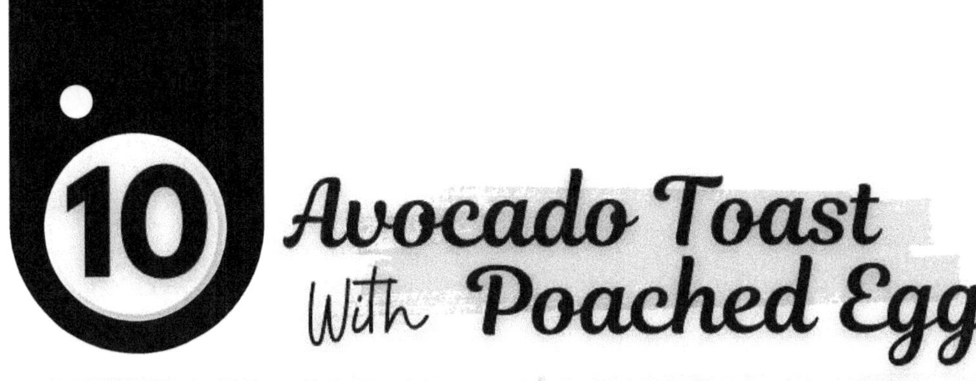

Avocado Toast with Poached Eggs

Introduction

Enjoy a delicious and nutritious breakfast with this avocado toast topped with poached eggs. Perfect for individuals in Stage 3 of diverticulitis maintenance and prevention, this recipe is packed with healthy fats, protein, and fiber to support digestive health and overall well-being. With creamy avocado, perfectly poached eggs, and whole grain toast, this breakfast is sure to become a favorite.

Ingredients

- 2 slices whole grain bread, toasted
- 1 ripe avocado, mashed
- 2 large eggs
- Salt and pepper to taste
- Red pepper flakes or paprika for garnish (optional)
- Fresh herbs, such as cilantro or parsley, for garnish (optional)

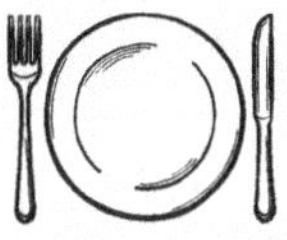

Prep Time	Cook Time	Serving
10 mins	5 mins	2

Preparation Method

1. While the bread is toasting, fill a saucepan with water and bring it to a gentle simmer over medium heat.
2. Crack one egg into a small bowl or ramekin.
3. Make a little whirlpool in the simmering water using a spoon.
4. Gently transfer the egg to the middle of the whirlpool.
5. Repeat with the second egg.
6. Poach the eggs for 3-4 minutes, or until the whites are set but the yolks are still runny.
7. Remove the poached eggs from the water using a slotted spoon and drain on a paper towel.
8. Spread the mashed avocado evenly onto the toasted bread slices.
9. Place a poached egg on top of each slice of avocado toast.
10. Season with salt, pepper, and red pepper flakes or paprika if desired.
11. Garnish with fresh herbs if desired.
12. Serve immediately and enjoy!

- Calories: 300 kcal
- Protein: 12g
- Fat: 20g
- Carbohydrates: 25g
- Fiber: 8g
- Sugar: 2g

Difficulty

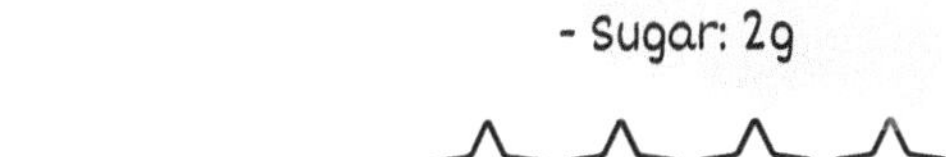

Rating

STAGE 3: MAINTENANCE AND PREVENTION RECIPE

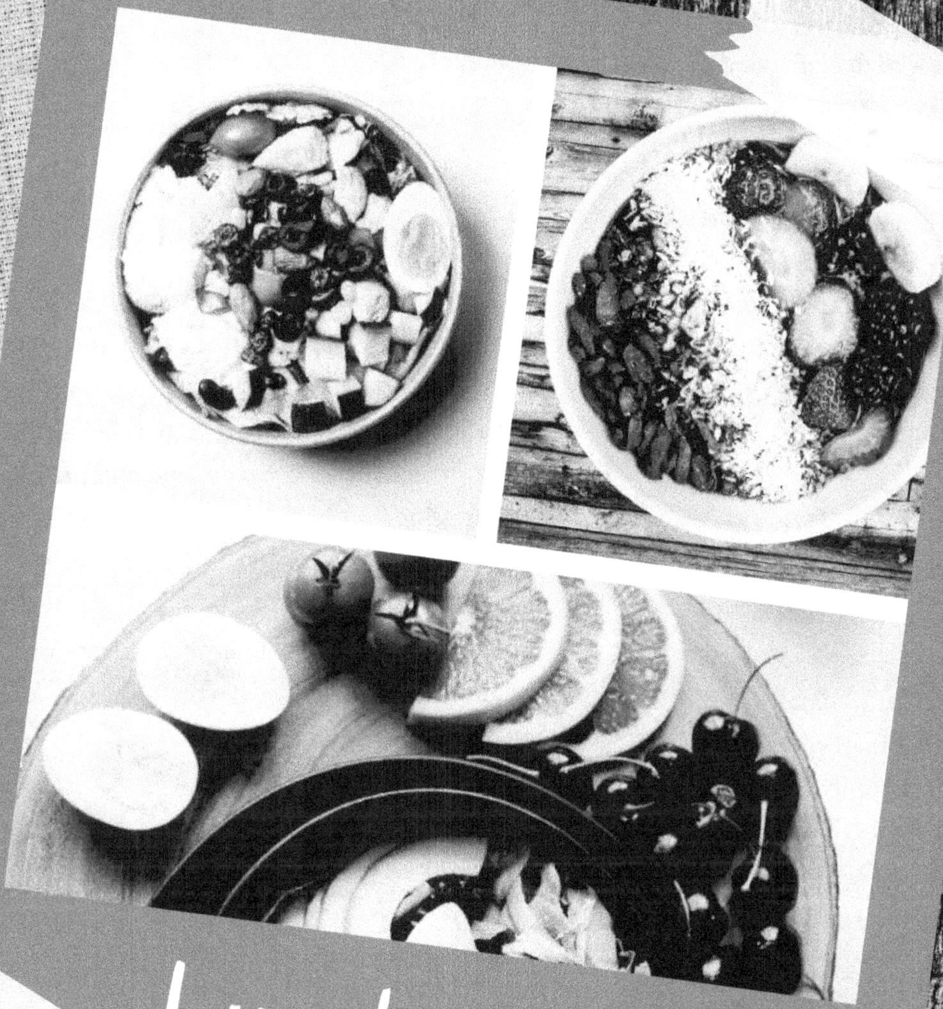

Lunch recipes

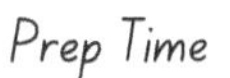

Prep Time

Cook Time

Rating

Difficulty

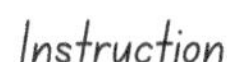

Instructions

Nutritional Value

Serving

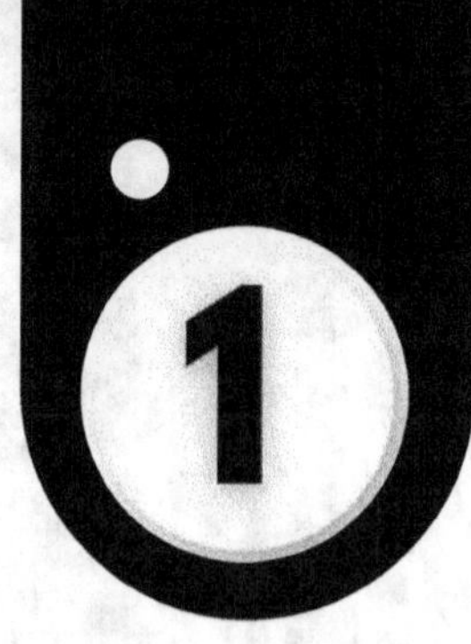

1 Mediterranean Chickpea Salad

Introduction

Indulge in the vibrant flavors of the Mediterranean with this refreshing chickpea salad. Packed with protein, fiber, and essential nutrients, this salad is perfect for individuals in Stage 3 of diverticulitis maintenance and prevention. With a combination of fresh vegetables, creamy feta cheese, and tangy vinaigrette, this salad is a delicious and satisfying meal option.

Ingredients

- 1 can (15 oz) chickpeas, drained and rinsed
- 1 cucumber, diced
- 1 bell pepper (any color), diced
- 1 cup cherry tomatoes, halved
- 1/4 red onion, thinly sliced
- 1/4 cup Kalamata olives, pitted and halved
- 2 oz feta cheese, crumbled
- 2 tablespoons fresh parsley, chopped
- 2 tablespoons extra virgin olive oil
- 1 tablespoon red wine vinegar
- 1 teaspoon dried oregano
- Salt and pepper to taste

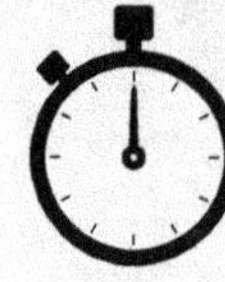

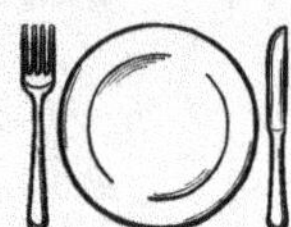

Prep Time 15 mins   **Cook Time** 30 mins   **Serving** 4

Preparation Method

1. In a large mixing bowl, combine the chickpeas, cucumber, bell pepper, cherry tomatoes, red onion, olives, feta cheese, and parsley.
2. In a small bowl, whisk together the olive oil, red wine vinegar, dried oregano, salt, and pepper to make the dressing.
3. Drizzle the salad with the dressing and gently mix to coat.
4. Let the salad marinate in the refrigerator for at least 30 minutes to allow the flavors to meld.
5. Serve chilled and enjoy!

- Calories: 250 kcal
- Protein: 8g
- Fat: 12g
- Carbohydrates: 30g
- Fiber: 8g
- Sugar: 5g

Difficulty

Rating

Grilled Veggie Wrap

Introduction

Enjoy a delicious and nutritious meal with this grilled veggie wrap. Packed with a variety of grilled vegetables, creamy hummus, and flavorful herbs, this wrap is perfect for individuals in Stage 3 of diverticulitis maintenance and prevention. With its satisfying texture and robust flavors, this wrap is sure to become a favorite lunch option.

Ingredients

- 1 large whole wheat or multigrain tortilla
- 1/4 cup hummus
- 1/2 cup mixed grilled vegetables (such as zucchini, bell peppers, eggplant, and onions), sliced
- 1/4 cup baby spinach or mixed greens
- 2 tablespoons crumbled feta cheese
- 1 tablespoon chopped fresh basil or parsley
- Salt and pepper to taste

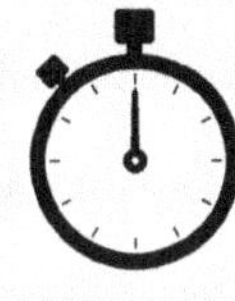  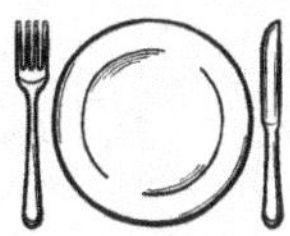

Prep Time
10 mins

Cook Time
10 mins
(for grilling vegetables)

Serving
1

Preparation Method

1. Spread the hummus evenly onto the tortilla.
2. Layer the grilled vegetables, baby spinach or mixed greens, crumbled feta cheese, and chopped herbs on top of the hummus.
3. Season with salt and pepper to your preferred taste.
4. Tightly roll up the tortilla, while also tucking in the edges/sides as you go.
5. Slice the wrap in half diagonally and secure with toothpicks if desired.
6. Serve immediately and enjoy!

- Calories: 300 kcal
- Protein: 8g
- Fat: 10g
- Carbohydrates: 45g
- Fiber: 8g
- Sugar: 5g

Difficulty

Rating

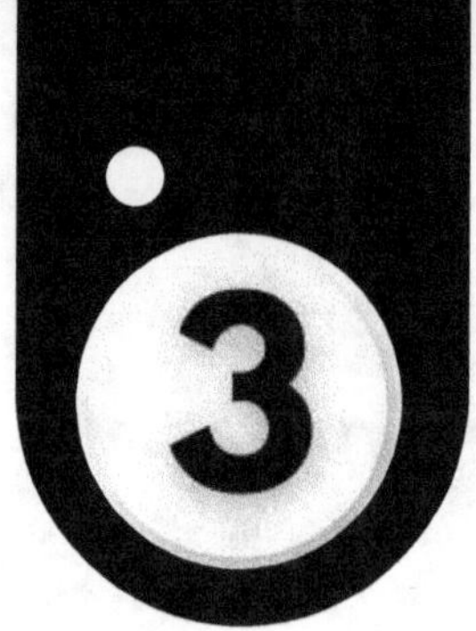

Turkey and Avocado BLT

Introduction

Indulge in a classic sandwich with a nutritious twist with this Turkey and Avocado BLT. Perfect for individuals in Stage 3 of diverticulitis maintenance and prevention, this sandwich is packed with protein, fiber, and healthy fats. With tender turkey slices, creamy avocado, crispy bacon, and fresh lettuce and tomato, this sandwich is sure to satisfy your taste buds while providing essential nutrients for digestive health.

Ingredients

- 2 slices whole grain bread, toasted
- 2-3 slices cooked turkey breast
- 2 slices cooked bacon
- 1/4 avocado, sliced
- 1 leaf lettuce
- 1 slice tomato
- 1 tablespoon mayonnaise
- Salt and pepper to taste

Prep Time
10 mins

Cook Time
10 mins
(for cooking bacon)

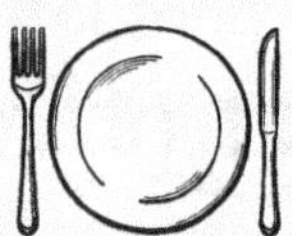

Serving
1

Preparation Method

1. Spread mayonnaise evenly onto one side of each toasted bread slice.
2. Layer the turkey breast, bacon slices, avocado slices, lettuce leaf, and tomato slice on one bread slice.
3. Season with salt and pepper to your preferred taste.
4. Top with the remaining bread slice to form a sandwich.
5. Cut the sandwich in half diagonally if desired.
6. Serve immediately and enjoy!

- Calories: 400 kcal
- Protein: 25g
- Fat: 20g
- Carbohydrates: 30g
- Fiber: 8g
- Sugar: 4g

Difficulty

Rating

Quinoa and Black Bean Salad

Introduction

Elevate your salad game with this flavorful and nutritious Quinoa and Black Bean Salad. Perfect for individuals in Stage 3 of diverticulitis maintenance and prevention, this salad is packed with protein, fiber, and essential nutrients to support digestive health and overall well-being. With fluffy quinoa, hearty black beans, crunchy vegetables, and zesty lime dressing, this salad is a satisfying and delicious meal option.

Ingredients

- 1/2 cup cooked quinoa, cooled
- 1/2 cup cooked black beans, drained and rinsed
- 1/4 cup diced bell pepper (any color)
- 1/4 cup diced cucumber
- 2 tablespoons chopped red onion
- 2 tablespoons chopped fresh cilantro
- 1 tablespoon extra virgin olive oil
- 1 tablespoon fresh lime juice
- 1/2 teaspoon ground cumin
- Salt and pepper to taste
- Optional toppings: avocado slices, cherry tomatoes, sliced jalapeños

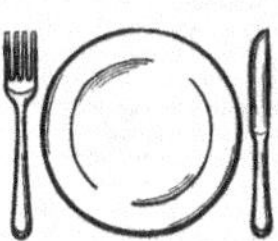

Prep Time 15 mins

Cook Time 15 mins (for cooking quinoa)

Serving 2

Preparation Method

1. In a large mixing bowl, combine the cooked quinoa, black beans, diced bell pepper, diced cucumber, chopped red onion, and chopped cilantro.
2. In a small bowl, whisk together the olive oil, lime juice, ground cumin, salt, and pepper to make the dressing.
3. Drizzle the salad with the dressing and gently mix to coat.
4. Taste and adjust seasoning if necessary.
5. Divide the salad into serving bowls and top with optional toppings if desired.
6. Serve chilled or at room temperature and enjoy!

- Calories: 300 kcal
- Protein: 10g
- Fat: 10g
- Carbohydrates: 40g
- Fiber: 8g
- Sugar: 2g

Difficulty

Rating

Tuna Salad Stuffed Bell Peppers

Introduction

Enjoy a light and refreshing meal with these Tuna Salad Stuffed Bell Peppers. Perfect for individuals in Stage 3 of diverticulitis maintenance and prevention, this dish is packed with protein, fiber, and essential nutrients. With tender bell peppers filled with a flavorful tuna salad mixture, this dish is both satisfying and nutritious.

Ingredients

- 2 large bell peppers (any color), halved and seeds removed
- 1 can (5 oz) tuna in water, drained
- 1/4 cup diced celery
- 1/4 cup diced red onion
- 2 tablespoons chopped fresh parsley
- 2 tablespoons mayonnaise
- 1 tablespoon lemon juice
- Salt and pepper to taste
- Optional toppings: sliced cherry tomatoes, avocado slices, chopped olives

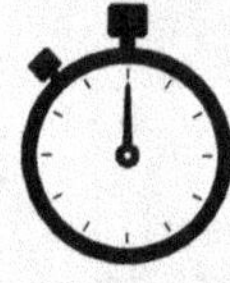  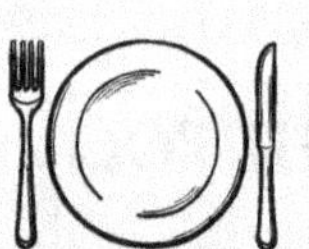

Prep Time 15 mins **Cook Time** 20-25 mins **Serving** 2

Preparation Method

1. Preheat the oven to 375°F (190°C).
2. Place the bell pepper halves on a baking sheet lined with parchment paper.
3. In a mixing bowl, combine the drained tuna, diced celery, diced red onion, chopped parsley, mayonnaise, lemon juice, salt, and pepper. Mix until well combined.
4. Spoon the tuna salad mixture into the bell pepper halves, dividing evenly.
5. Bake in the preheated oven for 20-25 minutes, or until the bell peppers are tender and slightly golden.
6. Take out of the oven and allow it to cool down for several minutes before serving.
7. Top with optional toppings if desired.
8. Serve warm or at room temperature and enjoy!

- Calories: 200 kcal
- Protein: 15g
- Fat: 10g
- Carbohydrates: 10g
- Fiber: 3g
- Sugar: 5g

Difficulty

Rating

Veggie and Hummus Plate

Introduction

Savor the flavors of fresh vegetables and creamy hummus with this Veggie and Hummus Plate. Perfect for individuals in Stage 3 of diverticulitis maintenance and prevention, this dish is packed with fiber, vitamins, and minerals to support digestive health. With a colorful assortment of vegetables and flavorful hummus, this plate is a nutritious and satisfying option for any meal.

Ingredients

- 1/2 cup baby carrots
- 1/2 cup cucumber slices
- 1/2 cup cherry tomatoes
- 1/2 cup bell pepper strips (any color)
- 1/4 cup sliced radishes
- 1/4 cup snap peas or sugar snap peas
- 1/4 cup hummus
- Optional garnishes: fresh herbs, black olives, lemon wedges

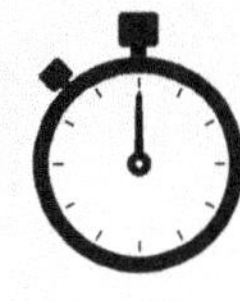 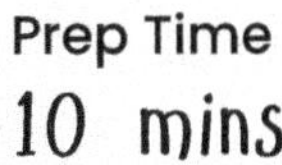  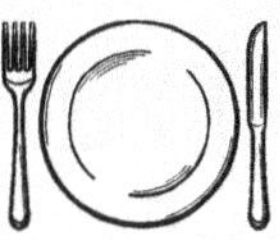

Prep Time 10 mins   **Cook Time** 0 mins   **Serving** 2

Preparation Method

1. Arrange the baby carrots, cucumber slices, cherry tomatoes, bell pepper strips, sliced radishes, and snap peas on a large plate or serving platter.
2. Place the hummus in the center of the plate.
3. Garnish with optional fresh herbs, black olives, or lemon wedges if desired.
4. Serve immediately and enjoy!

- Calories: 150 kcal
- Protein: 5g
- Fat: 7g
- Carbohydrates: 20g
- Fiber: 6g
- Sugar: 5g

Difficulty

Rating

Chicken and Quinoa Bowl

Introduction

Indulge in a wholesome and nutritious meal with this Chicken and Quinoa Bowl. Perfect for individuals in Stage 3 of diverticulitis maintenance and prevention, this dish is packed with lean protein, fiber-rich quinoa, and an assortment of colorful vegetables. With tender chicken breast, fluffy quinoa, and crunchy vegetables, this bowl is both satisfying and delicious.

Ingredients

- 1 cup cooked quinoa
- 1 grilled chicken breast, sliced
- 1/2 cup cherry tomatoes, halved
- 1/2 cup cucumber, diced
- 1/4 cup diced red onion
- 1/4 cup chopped fresh parsley
- 2 tablespoons lemon juice
- 1 tablespoon extra virgin olive oil
- Salt and pepper to taste
- Optional toppings: avocado slices, feta cheese crumbles, olives

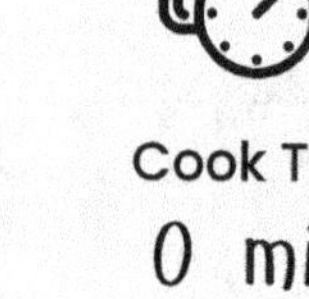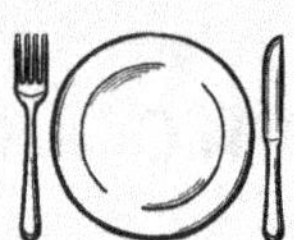

Prep Time
15 mins

Cook Time
0 mins
(for cooking quinoa
And grilled chicken)

Serving
2

Preparation Method

1. In a large mixing bowl, combine the cooked quinoa, sliced grilled chicken breast, cherry tomatoes, diced cucumber, diced red onion, and chopped fresh parsley.
2. In a small bowl, whisk together the lemon juice, extra virgin olive oil, salt, and pepper to make the dressing.
3. Pour the dressing over the quinoa and chicken mixture and toss gently to coat.
4. Taste and adjust seasoning if necessary.
5. Divide the mixture into serving bowls.
6. Top with optional toppings such as avocado slices, feta cheese crumbles, or olives if desired.
7. Serve immediately and enjoy!

- Calories: 350 kcal
- Protein: 25g
- Fat: 10g
- Carbohydrates: 40g
- Fiber: 6g
- Sugar: 3g

Difficulty

Rating

Salmon Salad Lettuce Wraps

Introduction

Enjoy a light and refreshing meal with these Salmon Salad Lettuce Wraps. Perfect for individuals in Stage 3 of diverticulitis maintenance and prevention, these wraps are packed with omega-3 fatty acids, protein, and an array of fresh vegetables. With flaky salmon, crunchy lettuce, and a tangy yogurt-dill dressing, these wraps are a healthy and satisfying option for any meal.

Prep Time
15 mins

Cook Time
15 mins
(for cooking salmon)

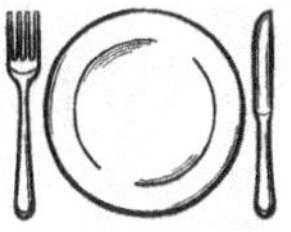

Serving
2

Ingredients

- 2 cooked salmon fillets, flaked
- 4 large lettuce leaves (such as butter or romaine)
- 1/2 cup diced cucumber
- 1/2 cup diced bell pepper (any color)
- 1/4 cup diced red onion
- 1/4 cup chopped fresh dill
- 1/4 cup plain Greek yogurt
- 1 tablespoon lemon juice
- Salt and pepper to taste
- Optional toppings: sliced avocado, cherry tomatoes, black olives

Preparation Method

1. In a large mixing bowl, combine the flaked cooked salmon, diced cucumber, diced bell pepper, diced red onion, chopped fresh dill, plain Greek yogurt, lemon juice, salt, and pepper.
2. Mix until well combined.
3. Spoon the salmon salad mixture onto each lettuce leaf.
4. Top with optional toppings such as sliced avocado, cherry tomatoes, or black olives if desired.
5. Fold the lettuce leaves over the filling to create wraps.
6. Serve immediately and enjoy!

- Calories: 250 kcal
- Protein: 20g
- Fat: 10g
- Carbohydrates: 15g
- Fiber: 4g
- Sugar: 5g

Difficulty

Rating

Lentil Soup
With Whole Grain Bread

Introduction

Warm up with a comforting bowl of Lentil Soup paired with wholesome Whole Grain Bread. This recipe is perfect for individuals in Stage 3 of diverticulitis maintenance and prevention, offering a hearty and nourishing meal packed with fiber, protein, and essential nutrients. With earthy lentils, vibrant vegetables, and hearty whole grain bread, this dish is both satisfying and nutritious.

Ingredients

- 1 cup dried green or brown lentils, rinsed and drained
- 4 cups vegetable broth
- 1 onion, diced
- 2 carrots, diced
- 2 celery stalks, diced
- 2 garlic cloves, minced
- 1 teaspoon dried thyme
- 1 teaspoon dried oregano
- 1 bay leaf
- Salt and pepper to taste
- Fresh parsley, chopped (for garnish)
- Whole grain bread, for serving

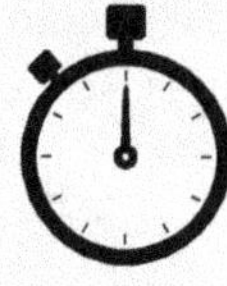

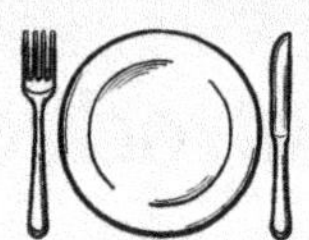

Prep Time 10 mins   **Cook Time** 40 mins   **Serving** 4

Preparation Method

1. One tablespoon of olive oil should be heated up over medium heat, using a large pot.
2. Add the diced onion, carrots, and celery to the pot and sauté until softened, about 5 minutes.
3. Add the minced garlic, dried thyme, and dried oregano to the pot and cook for another minute until fragrant.
4. Pour in the vegetable broth and add the rinsed lentils and bay leaf to the pot.
5. Bring the soup to a boil, then reduce the heat to low and simmer, covered, for about 30-40 minutes until the lentils are tender.
6. Season the soup with salt and pepper to your preferred taste.
7. Remove the bay leaf from the soup.
8. Ladle the soup into bowls, garnish with chopped fresh parsley, and serve hot with slices of whole grain bread.

- Calories: 250 kcal
- Protein: 15g
- Fat: 1g
- Carbohydrates: 45g
- Fiber: 15g
- Sugar: 5g

Difficulty

Rating

Veggie Sushi Rolls

Introduction

Experience the flavors of Japan with these delicious Veggie Sushi Rolls. Perfect for individuals in Stage 3 of diverticulitis maintenance and prevention, these rolls are packed with colorful vegetables, fiber-rich brown rice, and nutritious nori seaweed. With a delicate balance of flavors and textures, these sushi rolls are both satisfying and healthy.

Ingredients

- 2 cups cooked brown rice
- 4 nori seaweed sheets
- 1 cucumber, julienned
- 1 carrot, julienned
- 1 bell pepper, thinly sliced
- 1 avocado, sliced
- 1/4 cup pickled ginger
- 1/4 cup low-sodium soy sauce or tamari
- Wasabi and/or sriracha (optional)
- Bamboo sushi mat (for rolling)
- Sharp knife (for slicing)

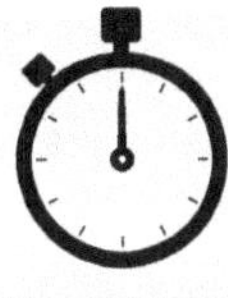  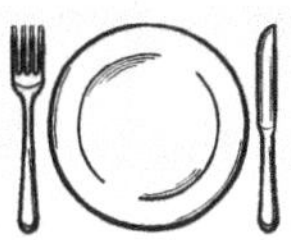

Prep Time 20 mins

Cook Time 30 mins (for cooking rice)

Serving 4

Preparation Method

1. Place a nori seaweed sheet shiny side down on a bamboo sushi mat.
2. Spread a thin layer of cooked brown rice evenly over the nori, leaving about a 1-inch border at the top edge.
3. Arrange the julienned cucumber, carrot, bell pepper, avocado, and pickled ginger in a line across the center of the rice.
4. Starting from the bottom edge, tightly roll the sushi using the bamboo mat, pressing gently to seal.
5. Wet the top edge of the nori with a little water to help seal the roll.
6. Repeat with the remaining nori sheets and ingredients.
7. Cut each sushi roll into bite-sized pieces using a sharp knife.
8. Serve the sushi rolls with low-sodium soy sauce or tamari for dipping, and wasabi and/or sriracha if desired.

- Calories: 200 kcal
- Protein: 5g
- Fat: 5g
- Carbohydrates: 35g
- Fiber: 8g
- Sugar: 4g

Difficulty

Rating

STAGE 3: MAINTENANCE AND PREVENTION RECIPE

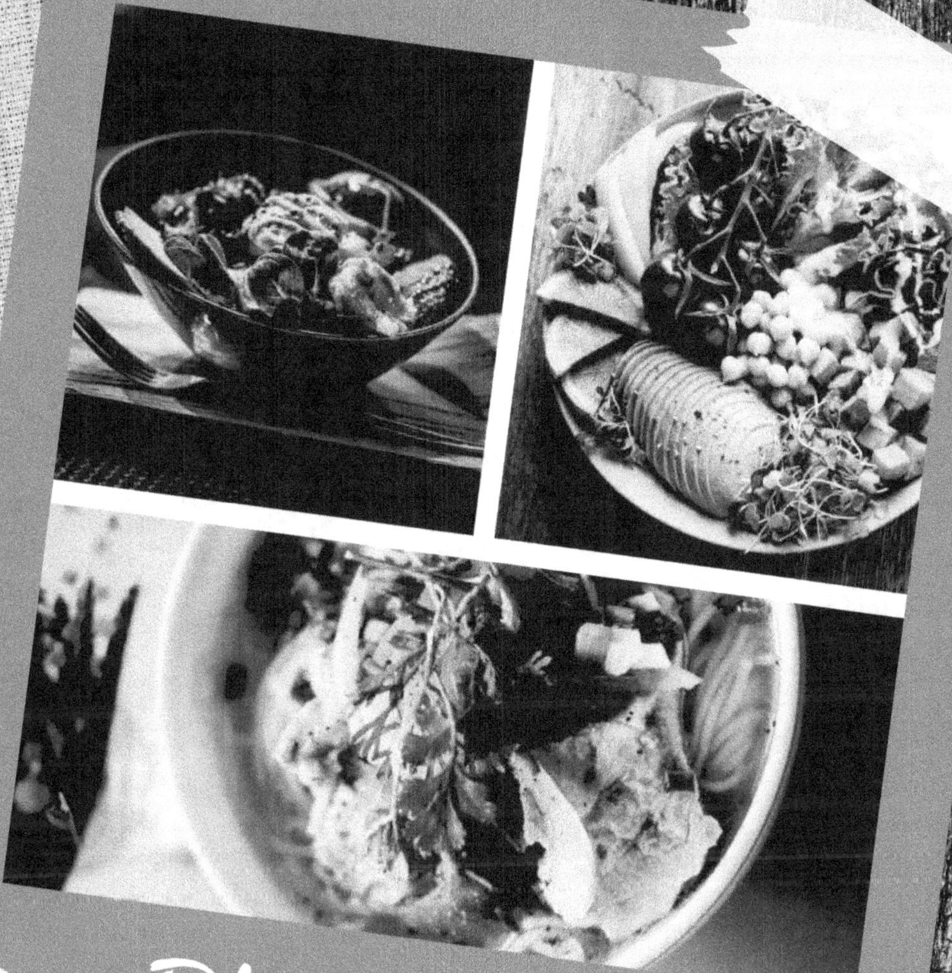

Dinner recipes

Prep Time

Cook Time

Rating

Difficulty

Instructions

Nutritional Value

Serving

Lemon Garlic Salmon

Introduction

Indulge in the vibrant flavors of Lemon Garlic Salmon, a delicious and nutritious dish perfect for Stage 3 of diverticulitis maintenance and prevention. This recipe features tender salmon fillets marinated in a zesty lemon and garlic sauce, then baked to perfection. Packed with omega-3 fatty acids and protein, this dish is both satisfying and beneficial for overall health.

Ingredients

- 4 salmon fillets (6 oz each)
- 2 cloves garlic, minced
- Zest and juice of 1 lemon
- 2 tablespoons olive oil
- 1 tablespoon chopped fresh parsley
- Salt and pepper to taste
- Lemon slices for garnish

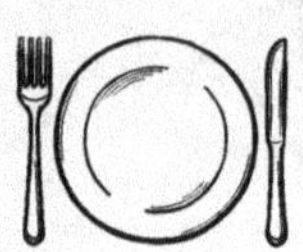

Prep Time
10 mins

Cook Time
12-15 mins

Serving
4

Preparation Method

1. Preheat your oven to 375°F (190°C), then line a baking sheet with parchment paper.

2. In a small bowl, whisk together the minced garlic, lemon zest, lemon juice, olive oil, chopped parsley, salt, and pepper.

3. Place the salmon fillets on the prepared baking sheet and brush the lemon garlic mixture over each fillet, coating evenly.

4. Arrange lemon slices on top of each fillet for additional flavor.

5. Bake the salmon in the preheated oven for 12-15 minutes, or until the fish is cooked through and flakes easily with a fork.

6. Take the salmon out of the oven and allow it rest for a few minutes before serving.

7. Garnish with additional chopped parsley and lemon slices if desired.

8. Serve the Lemon Garlic Salmon hot with your favorite side dishes, such as steamed vegetables or quinoa.

- Calories: 300 kcal
- Protein: 25g
- Fat: 20g
- Carbohydrates: 2g
- Fiber: 0g
- Sugar: 0g

Difficulty

Rating

② Turkey Meatloaf With Mashed Cauliflower

Introduction

Enjoy a comforting and wholesome meal with Turkey Meatloaf paired with creamy Mashed Cauliflower, ideal for Stage 3 of diverticulitis maintenance and prevention. This recipe features lean ground turkey seasoned with herbs and spices, baked to perfection and served alongside silky mashed cauliflower. Packed with protein and fiber, this dish is both satisfying and nutritious.

Ingredients

For the Turkey Meatloaf:
- 1 lb lean ground turkey
- 1/2 cup breadcrumbs (whole grain or gluten-free)
- 1/4 cup milk (dairy or non-dairy)
- 1 egg
- 1/4 cup finely chopped onion
  2 cloves garlic, minced
- 1 teaspoon dried oregano
- 1 teaspoon dried thyme
- Salt and pepper to taste
- 1/4 cup ketchup or tomato sauce (optional, for topping)

For the Mashed Cauliflower:
- 1 head cauliflower, chopped into florets
- 2 cloves garlic
- 2 tablespoons butter or olive oil
- Salt and pepper to taste
- Chopped fresh parsley for garnish

  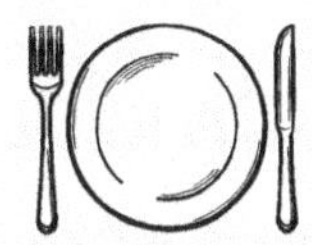

Prep Time	Cook Time	Serving
20 mins	45–50 mins	4

Preparation Method

For the Turkey Meatloaf:

1. Preheat the oven to 375°F (190°C) and lightly grease a loaf pan with cooking spray.

2. In a large mixing bowl, combine the ground turkey, breadcrumbs, milk, egg, chopped onion, minced garlic, dried oregano, dried thyme, salt, and pepper. Mix until well combined.

3. Transfer the turkey mixture to the prepared loaf pan and shape it into a loaf.

4. If desired, spread a thin layer of ketchup or tomato sauce over the top of the meatloaf.

5. Bake the turkey meatloaf in the preheated oven for 45-50 minutes, or until cooked through and golden brown on top.

6. Remove the meatloaf from the oven and let it rest for a few minutes before slicing.

For the Mashed Cauliflower:

1. While the meatloaf is baking, steam the cauliflower florets and garlic cloves until tender, about 10-12 minutes.

2. Drain the steamed cauliflower and garlic, then transfer them to a food processor.

3. Add the butter or olive oil to the food processor and season with salt and pepper to taste.

4. Pulse the mixture until smooth and creamy, scraping down the sides of the processor as needed.

5. Taste and adjust seasoning if necessary.

6. Transfer the mashed cauliflower to a serving dish and garnish with chopped fresh parsley.

- Calories: 250 kcal (meatloaf only) + 100 kcal (mashed cauliflower)
- Protein: 20g (meatloaf only) + 5g (mashed cauliflower)
- Fat: 10g (meatloaf only) + 5g (mashed cauliflower)
- Carbohydrates: 15g (meatloaf only) + 10g (mashed cauliflower)
- Fiber: 3g (meatloaf only) + 5g (mashed cauliflower)
- Sugar: 3g (meatloaf only) + 3g (mashed cauliflower)

Difficulty

Rating

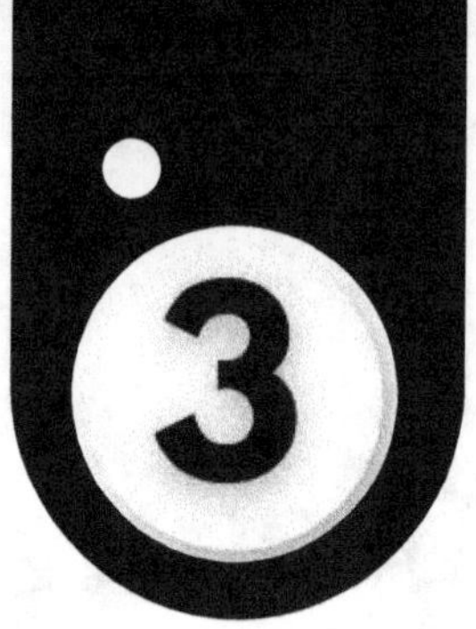

Stuffed Acorn Squash

Introduction

Delight your taste buds with Stuffed Acorn Squash, a nutritious and flavorful dish perfect for Stage 3 of diverticulitis maintenance and prevention. This recipe features tender roasted acorn squash halves filled with a delicious mixture of quinoa, vegetables, and herbs. Packed with fiber, vitamins, and minerals, this dish is both satisfying and nourishing.

Ingredients

- 2 acorn squash, halved and seeds removed
- 1 cup quinoa, rinsed
- 2 cups vegetable broth
- 1 tablespoon olive oil
- 1 onion, diced
- 2 cloves garlic, minced
- 1 bell pepper, diced
- 1 zucchini, diced
- 1 cup cherry tomatoes, halved
- 1 teaspoon dried thyme
- 1 teaspoon dried oregano
- Salt and pepper to taste
- Fresh parsley for garnish

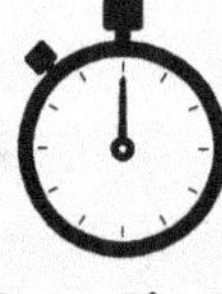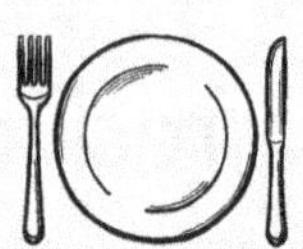

Prep Time	Cook Time	Serving
15 mins	45 mins	4

Preparation Method

1. Preheat the oven to 400°F (200°C) and line a baking sheet with parchment paper.
2. Place the acorn squash halves on the prepared baking sheet, cut side down, and roast in the preheated oven for 30-35 minutes, or until tender.
3. In the meantime, prepare the quinoa. Bring the vegetable broth to a boil in a medium-sized saucepan. Stir in the quinoa, reduce heat to low, cover, and simmer for 15-20 minutes, or until the quinoa is cooked and fluffy.
4. The olive oil should be heated up over medium heat, using a large skillet. Add in the chopped onion and cook for about 3–4 minutes, or until it's soft and tender.
5. Add the minced garlic, diced bell pepper, and diced zucchini to the skillet. Cook for an additional 5-6 minutes, or until the vegetables are tender.
6. Stir in the cooked quinoa, cherry tomatoes, dried thyme, dried oregano, salt, and pepper. To ensure it is well cooked, cook for a further two to three minutes.
7. Once the acorn squash halves are tender, remove them from the oven and carefully flip them over.
8. Spoon the quinoa and vegetable mixture into each squash half, filling them generously.
9. Return the stuffed acorn squash to the oven and bake for an additional 10 minutes to heat through.
10. Remove from the oven and garnish with fresh parsley before serving.

- Calories: 300 kcal
- Protein: 8g
- Fat: 6g
- Carbohydrates: 55g
- Fiber: 10g
- Sugar: 7g

Difficulty

Rating

Mediterranean Chicken Skewers

Introduction

Transport your taste buds to the Mediterranean with these flavorful Chicken Skewers, a delightful dish perfect for Stage 3 of diverticulitis maintenance and prevention. This recipe features tender chunks of chicken marinated in a zesty blend of Mediterranean spices, threaded onto skewers with colorful vegetables, and grilled to perfection. Packed with protein and antioxidants, these skewers are both delicious and nutritious.

Ingredients

- 1 lb boneless, skinless chicken breasts, cut into cubes
- 1 bell pepper, cut into chunks
- 1 red onion, cut into chunks
- 1 zucchini, sliced
- 1/4 cup olive oil
- 2 tablespoons lemon juice
- 2 cloves garlic, minced
- 1 teaspoon dried oregano
- 1 teaspoon dried thyme
- 1 teaspoon paprika
- Salt and pepper to taste
- Wooden skewers, soaked in water for 30 minutes

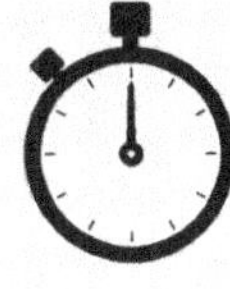

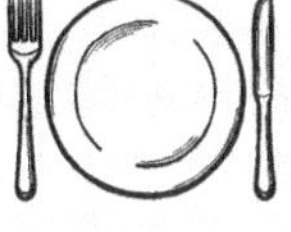

Prep Time	Cook Time	Serving
15 mins	10-12 mins	4
(plus marinating time)		

Preparation Method

1. In a large bowl, whisk together the olive oil, lemon juice, minced garlic, dried oregano, dried thyme, paprika, salt, and pepper to create the marinade.

2. Add the cubed chicken breast to the marinade and toss until evenly coated. To marinate, cover and chill for at least half an hour(30 minutes).

3. Preheat the grill to medium-high heat.

4. Thread the marinated chicken cubes, bell pepper chunks, red onion chunks, and zucchini slices onto the soaked wooden skewers, alternating between the chicken and vegetables.

5. Grill the skewers on the hot grill for about 10-12 minutes, flipping regularly, or until the chicken is fully cooked and the veggies are soft and gently browned.

6. Remove the skewers from the grill and let them rest for a few minutes before serving.

7. Serve the Mediterranean Chicken Skewers hot with your favorite side dishes, such as rice, couscous, or a Greek salad.

- Calories: 250 kcal
- Protein: 25g
- Fat: 12g
- Carbohydrates: 10g
- Fiber: 3g
- Sugar: 4g

Difficulty

Rating

Cauliflower Fried Rice

Introduction

Enjoy a healthier twist on a classic favorite with Cauliflower Fried Rice, a nutritious and delicious dish perfect for Stage 3 of diverticulitis maintenance and prevention. This recipe replaces traditional rice with finely chopped cauliflower, offering a low-carb, gluten-free alternative packed with vitamins and minerals. Combined with colorful vegetables and savory seasonings, this cauliflower fried rice is sure to satisfy your cravings without compromising your health.

Ingredients

- - 1 medium head cauliflower
- 2 tablespoons olive oil
- 2 cloves garlic, minced
- 1 onion, diced
- 2 carrots, diced
- 1 cup frozen peas
- 2 eggs, beaten
- 3 tablespoons soy sauce (or tamari for gluten-free)
- 1 teaspoon sesame oil
- Salt and pepper to taste
- Green onions, sliced (for garnish)

 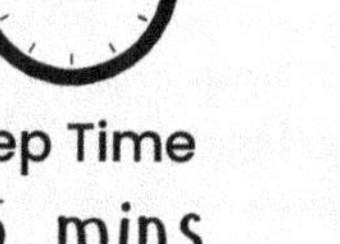  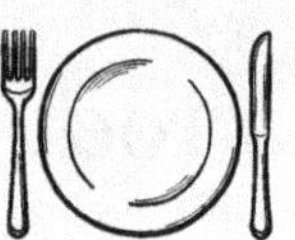

Prep Time 15 mins **Cook Time** 15 mins **Serving** 4

Preparation Method

1. Wash the cauliflower and remove the leaves and stem. Then the cauliflower should be chopped into florets and put in a food processor. Pulse until the cauliflower resembles rice-sized pieces.

2. Heat 1 tablespoon of olive oil in a large skillet or wok over medium heat. Add the chopped onion and minced garlic, and sauté until transparent and aromatic.

3. Add the diced carrots to the skillet and cook for a few minutes until slightly softened.

4. Push the vegetables to one side of the skillet and add the beaten eggs to the empty side. Scramble the eggs until cooked through, then mix them with the vegetables.

5. Add the remaining tablespoon of olive oil to the skillet, then stir in the riced cauliflower and frozen peas. Cook the cauliflower for about five to seven minutes, stirring now and again, until it becomes soft.

6. Drizzle the soy sauce and sesame oil over the cauliflower fried rice, and season with salt and pepper to taste. Stir well to combine.

7. Cook for a further 2-3 minutes, allowing the flavors to blend in together.

8. Remove from heat and garnish with sliced green onions before serving

- Calories: 150 kcal
- Protein: 6g
- Fat: 8g
- Carbohydrates: 15g
- Fiber: 5g
- Sugar: 5g

Difficulty

**Rating

Spinach With Mushroom Stuffed Chicken

Introduction

Indulge in a gourmet meal with Spinach and Mushroom Stuffed Chicken, a flavorful and elegant dish perfect for Stage 3 of diverticulitis maintenance and prevention. This recipe features tender chicken breasts stuffed with a savory mixture of sautéed spinach, mushrooms, garlic, and cheese, creating a deliciously satisfying entrée that's sure to impress. Serve with your preferred side dishes for a filling and well-rounded dinner.

Ingredients

- 4 boneless, skinless chicken breasts
- Salt and pepper to taste
- 1 tablespoon olive oil
- 2 cups fresh spinach leaves
- 1 cup mushrooms, sliced
- 2 cloves garlic, minced
- 1/2 cup shredded mozzarella cheese
- 1/4 cup grated Parmesan cheese
- 1 teaspoon dried Italian herbs
- Toothpicks (for securing)

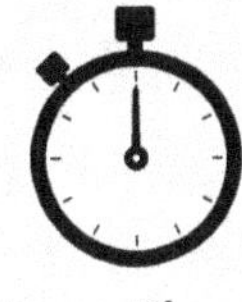

Prep Time
20 mins

Cook Time
30 mins

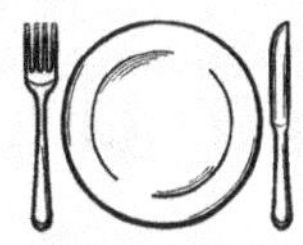

Serving
4

Preparation Method

1. Lightly butter a baking dish and preheat the oven to 375°F (190°C).
2. Place the chicken breasts between two sheets of plastic wrap and gently pound them to an even thickness. Season both sides with salt and pepper to your preferred taste.
3. The olive oil should be heated up over medium heat, using a large skillet. Add the minced garlic and sauté until fragrant, about 1 minute.
4. Add the sliced mushrooms to the skillet and cook until they release their moisture and become golden brown, about 5-7 minutes.
5. Add the fresh spinach leaves to the skillet and cook until wilted, about 2-3 minutes. Remove from the heat and set aside to get cool slightly.
6. In a mixing bowl, combine the sautéed spinach and mushrooms with the shredded mozzarella cheese, grated Parmesan cheese, and dried Italian herbs. Mix until well combined.
7. Place a spoonful of the spinach and mushroom mixture onto each chicken breast. Roll up the chicken breasts tightly and secure with toothpicks to hold the filling in place.
8. Place the stuffed chicken breasts in the prepared baking dish and bake in the preheated oven for 25-30 minutes, or until the chicken is cooked through and the filling is hot and bubbly.
9. Remove from the oven and let the chicken rest for a few minutes before serving.
10. Serve the Spinach and Mushroom Stuffed Chicken hot with your favorite side dishes, such as roasted vegetables or a salad.

- Calories: 250 kcal
- Protein: 30g
- Fat: 10g
- Carbohydrates: 5g
- Fiber: 2g
- Sugar: 2g

Difficulty

Rating

Baked Eggplant Rollatini

Introduction

Elevate your dinner with Baked Eggplant Rollatini, a flavorful and elegant dish perfect for Stage 3 of diverticulitis maintenance and prevention. Thin slices of eggplant are filled with a savory mixture of ricotta cheese, spinach, and herbs, then rolled up and baked to perfection with marinara sauce and melted cheese. This vegetarian entree is both satisfying and nutritious, making it a delightful addition to any meal.

Ingredients

-- 2 medium eggplants
- Salt
- 1 cup ricotta cheese
- 1 cup shredded mozzarella cheese, divided
- 1/4 cup grated Parmesan cheese, plus extra for topping
- 1 egg, lightly beaten
- 1 cup chopped spinach, cooked and drained
- 2 cloves garlic, minced
- 1 teaspoon dried Italian herbs
- 2 cups marinara sauce
- Fresh basil leaves, for garnish

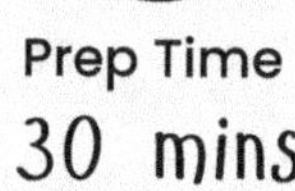

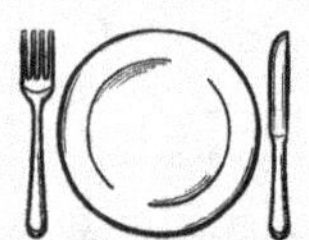

Prep Time	Cook Time	Serving
30 mins	30 mins	4

Preparation Method

1. Grease a baking dish lightly and preheat the oven to 375°F (190°C).
2. Slice the eggplants lengthwise into thin strips, about 1/4-inch thick. Place the slices on a baking sheet and sprinkle both sides with salt. Let them sit for 10-15 minutes to release excess moisture, then pat dry with paper towels.
3. In a mixing bowl, combine the ricotta cheese, 1/2 cup of shredded mozzarella cheese, grated Parmesan cheese, beaten egg, chopped spinach, minced garlic, and dried Italian herbs. Mix until well combined.
4. Spread a thin layer of marinara sauce on the bottom of the prepared baking dish.
5. Place a spoonful of the ricotta mixture onto each eggplant slice and spread it evenly. Roll up the eggplant slices and place them seam-side down in the baking dish.
6. Pour the remaining marinara sauce over the eggplant rollatini, then sprinkle the remaining shredded mozzarella cheese and extra grated Parmesan cheese on top.
7. Cover the baking dish with aluminum foil and bake in the preheated oven for 25-30 minutes, or until the cheese is melted and bubbly.
8. Remove the foil and broil for an additional 2-3 minutes, until the cheese is golden brown.
9. Just before serving, garnish with fresh basil leaves.

- Calories: 300 kcal
- Protein: 15g
- Fat: 15g
- Carbohydrates: 25g
- Fiber: 10g
- Sugar: 10g

Difficulty

Rating

Baked Eggplant Rollatini

Introduction

Elevate your dinner with Baked Eggplant Rollatini, a flavorful and elegant dish perfect for Stage 3 of diverticulitis maintenance and prevention. Thin slices of eggplant are filled with a savory mixture of ricotta cheese, spinach, and herbs, then rolled up and baked to perfection with marinara sauce and melted cheese. This vegetarian entree is both satisfying and nutritious, making it a delightful addition to any meal.

Ingredients

-- 2 medium eggplants
- Salt
- 1 cup ricotta cheese
- 1 cup shredded mozzarella cheese, divided
- 1/4 cup grated Parmesan cheese, plus extra for topping
- 1 egg, lightly beaten
- 1 cup chopped spinach, cooked and drained
- 2 cloves garlic, minced
- 1 teaspoon dried Italian herbs
- 2 cups marinara sauce
- Fresh basil leaves, for garnish

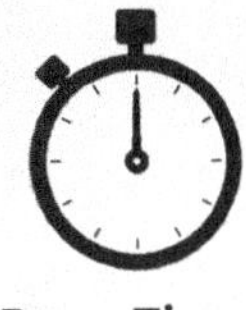

Prep Time
30 mins

Cook Time
30 mins

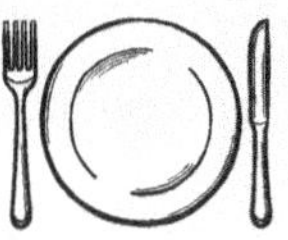

Serving
4

Preparation Method

1. Grease a baking dish lightly and preheat the oven to 375°F (190°C).
2. Slice the eggplants lengthwise into thin strips, about 1/4-inch thick. Place the slices on a baking sheet and sprinkle both sides with salt. Let them sit for 10-15 minutes to release excess moisture, then pat dry with paper towels.
3. In a mixing bowl, combine the ricotta cheese, 1/2 cup of shredded mozzarella cheese, grated Parmesan cheese, beaten egg, chopped spinach, minced garlic, and dried Italian herbs. Mix until well combined.
4. Spread a thin layer of marinara sauce on the bottom of the prepared baking dish.
5. Place a spoonful of the ricotta mixture onto each eggplant slice and spread it evenly. Roll up the eggplant slices and place them seam-side down in the baking dish.
6. Pour the remaining marinara sauce over the eggplant rollatini, then sprinkle the remaining shredded mozzarella cheese and extra grated Parmesan cheese on top.
7. Cover the baking dish with aluminum foil and bake in the preheated oven for 25-30 minutes, or until the cheese is melted and bubbly.
8. Remove the foil and broil for an additional 2-3 minutes, until the cheese is golden brown.
9. Just before serving, garnish with fresh basil leaves.

- Calories: 300 kcal
- Protein: 15g
- Fat: 15g
- Carbohydrates: 25g
- Fiber: 10g
- Sugar: 10g

Difficulty

Rating

Roasted Vegetable Frittata

Introduction

Savor the delightful flavors of Roasted Vegetable Frittata, a nutritious and versatile dish perfect for Stage 3 of diverticulitis maintenance and prevention. This hearty frittata features a colorful array of roasted vegetables, eggs, and cheese, baked to golden perfection. Whether enjoyed for breakfast, brunch, or dinner, this frittata is a satisfying meal option that can be customized with your favorite vegetables and herbs.

Ingredients

- 1 tablespoon olive oil
- 1 onion, diced
- 1 bell pepper, diced
- 1 zucchini, diced
- 1 cup cherry tomatoes, halved
- 1 cup spinach leaves
- 8 large eggs
- 1/4 cup milk (or dairy-free alternative)
- 1/2 cup shredded cheese (such as cheddar or mozzarella)
- Salt and pepper to taste
- Fresh herbs for garnish (optional)

  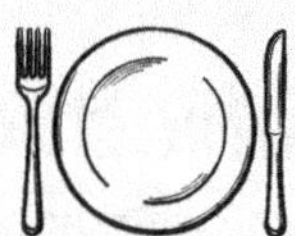

Prep Time 15 mins **Cook Time** 25 mins **Serving** 6

Preparation Method

1. Preheat the oven to 375°F (190°C). Lightly grease a 9-inch pie dish or oven-safe skillet.

2. The olive oil should be heated up over medium heat, using a large skillet. Add the diced onion and bell pepper, and cook until softened, about 5 minutes.

3. Add the diced zucchini and cherry tomatoes to the skillet. Cook for an additional 3 - 4 minutes, or until the vegetables are soft and tender.

4. Add the spinach leaves to the skillet and cook until wilted, about 2 minutes. Remove from heat and set aside.

5. In a mixing bowl, whisk together the eggs, milk, shredded cheese, salt, and pepper until well combined.

6. Pour the egg mixture into the prepared pie dish or skillet. Add the cooked vegetables on top, distributing them evenly.

7. Place the dish or skillet in the preheated oven and bake for 20-25 minutes, or until the frittata is set in the center and lightly golden on top.

8. Take it out of the oven and let it cool down a few minutes before slicing.

9. Garnish with fresh herbs if desired, then slice and serve the Roasted Vegetable Frittata warm or at room temperature.

- Calories: 180 kcal
- Protein: 12g
- Fat: 11g
- Carbohydrates: 8g
- Fiber: 2g
- Sugar: 3g

Difficulty

Rating

Eggplant Parmesan

Introduction

Indulge in the comforting flavors of Eggplant Parmesan, a wholesome dish perfect for Stage 3 of diverticulitis maintenance and prevention. This classic Italian-inspired recipe features tender slices of eggplant layered with marinara sauce, melted cheese, and aromatic herbs. Baked to golden perfection, Eggplant Parmesan is a hearty and satisfying meal that will delight your taste buds while supporting your digestive health.

Ingredients

- 2 large eggplants, sliced into 1/2-inch rounds
- Salt
- 2 cups marinara sauce
- 1 cup shredded mozzarella cheese
- 1/2 cup grated Parmesan cheese
- 1/4 cup chopped fresh basil
- 1/4 cup chopped fresh parsley
- 1/2 cup breadcrumbs (optional)
- Olive oil, for brushing

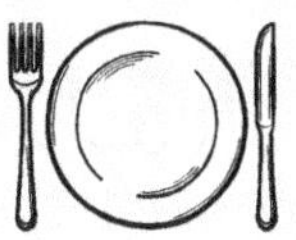

Prep Time
30 mins

Cook Time
45 mins

Serving
6

Preparation Method

1. Preheat the oven to 375°F (190°C). Line your baking sheet with a parchment paper.
2. Put the slices of eggplant in a colander and season with salt. Let them sit for 20-30 minutes to draw out excess moisture. After giving the eggplant slices a quick rinse in cold water, blot them dry with paper towels.
3. Place the eggplant slices on the baking sheet that has been prepared. Apply a thin layer of olive oil on both sides of every slice.
4. Bake the eggplant slices in the preheated oven for 15-20 minutes, or until they are tender and slightly golden.
5. Brush the bottom of a baking dish with a thin coating of marinara sauce. Place slices of baked eggplant on top in a layer.
6. Sprinkle some shredded mozzarella and grated Parmesan cheese over the eggplant slices. Add a sprinkle of chopped basil and parsley.
7. Repeat the layers until all the ingredients are used, ending with a layer of cheese and herbs on top.
8. If desired, sprinkle breadcrumbs over the top layer for added texture.
9. Cover the baking dish with aluminum foil and bake in the oven for 25-30 minutes, or until the cheese is melted and bubbly.
10. Remove the foil and bake for an additional 5-10 minutes, or until the top is golden brown.
11. Remove from the oven and let it cool for a few minutes before serving.

- Calories: 250 kcal
- Protein: 12g
- Fat: 10g
- Carbohydrates: 30g
- Fiber: 8g
- Sugar: 12g

Difficulty

**Rating

Baked Cod with Herb Crust

Introduction

Savor the delicate flavors of Baked Cod with Herb Crust, a nutritious and delicious dish perfect for Stage 3 of diverticulitis maintenance and prevention. This simple yet elegant recipe features fresh cod fillets coated in a flavorful herb crust, baked to tender perfection. With a burst of aromatic herbs and zesty lemon, this baked cod dish is sure to become a favorite in your healthy eating repertoire.

Ingredients

- 4 cod fillets (about 6 ounces each)
- Salt and pepper to taste
- 1 tablespoon olive oil
- 1/4 cup breadcrumbs
- 2 tablespoons chopped fresh parsley
- 1 tablespoon chopped fresh dill
- 1 tablespoon chopped fresh chives
- 1 tablespoon grated Parmesan cheese
- 1 clove garlic, minced
- Zest of 1 lemon
- Lemon wedges, for serving

 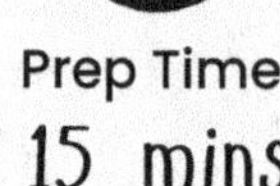  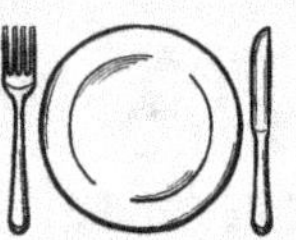

Prep Time 15 mins

Cook Time 15 mins

Serving 4

Preparation Method

1. Preheat the oven to 400°F (200°C). Apply a little application of olive oil to your baking dish.

2. Season the cod fillets with salt and pepper on both sides, then place them in the prepared baking dish.

3. In a small bowl, combine the breadcrumbs, chopped parsley, dill, chives, grated Parmesan cheese, minced garlic, and lemon zest. Mix well to combine.

4. Drizzle the olive oil over the seasoned cod fillets, then press the herb breadcrumb mixture evenly onto the top of each fillet, coating them generously.

5. Bake the cod fillets in the preheated oven for 12-15 minutes, or until the fish is opaque and flakes easily with a fork.

6. Take it out of the oven and give it some time to settle before serving.

7. Serve the Baked Cod with Herb Crust with lemon wedges on the side for squeezing over the fish.

- Calories: 220 kcal
- Protein: 25g
- Fat: 7g
- Carbohydrates: 10g
- Fiber: 1g
- Sugar: 1g

Difficulty

Rating

Chapter 4

Dining Out and Special Occasions

Navigating dining out and special occasions while following a diverticulitis diet can present its challenges, but with some thoughtful planning and smart strategies, you can still enjoy delicious meals and participate fully in social gatherings and travel experiences.

Making Informed Choices at Restaurants:

When dining out, it's essential to make informed choices that align with your diverticulitis diet. Here are some tips to help you navigate restaurant menus:

1. Research the Menu in Advance: Many restaurants now offer their menus online, allowing you to review the options beforehand. Look for dishes that include lean proteins, cooked vegetables, and whole grains.

2. Customize Your Order: Don't hesitate to ask your server for modifications to suit your dietary needs. Request grilled or baked proteins instead of fried, and ask for sauces and dressings on the side to control the amount you consume.

3. Choose Fiber-Rich Options: Opt for dishes that are rich in fiber, such as salads with leafy greens, beans, and vegetables. These can help promote healthy digestion and prevent flare-ups of diverticulitis.

4. Be Mindful of Portions: Restaurant servings are often larger than what you would eat at home. Consider sharing an entree with a dining companion or ask for a to-go box to portion out your meal before you start eating.

5. Limit Trigger Foods: Avoid foods that may trigger diverticulitis symptoms, such as spicy dishes, high-fat foods, and those containing seeds or nuts.

Strategies for Social Gatherings and Travel:

Maintaining your diverticulitis diet during social gatherings and travel requires some extra planning and flexibility. Below are some strategies and techniques that will help you stay on track:

1. Plan Ahead: If you know you'll be attending a social event or traveling, plan your meals and snacks accordingly. Pack portable, diverticulitis-friendly snacks like nuts, seeds, plain yogurt, and fruit to have on hand.

2. Communicate Your Needs: Don't be afraid to communicate your dietary needs to hosts or travel companions. Let them know about your condition and any specific foods you need to avoid.

3. BYO Dish: Offer to bring a dish to social gatherings, ensuring there's something diverticulitis-friendly for you to enjoy. Prepare a nutrient-rich salad, vegetable platter, or lean protein option that aligns with your dietary requirements.

4. Scope Out Local Options: When traveling, research nearby restaurants or grocery stores that offer diverticulitis-friendly options. Look for places that serve grilled proteins, steamed vegetables, and whole grains.

5. Stay Hydrated: Remember to drink plenty of water, especially when traveling. Dehydration can exacerbate digestive issues, so aim to stay hydrated throughout the day.

By making informed choices at restaurants and implementing smart strategies for social gatherings and travel, you can continue to enjoy delicious meals and participate in special occasions while managing your diverticulitis effectively. Remember to prioritize your health and well-being, and don't hesitate to advocate for yourself and your dietary needs.

Chapter 5
Tips for Long-Term Success

During the acute phase of diverticulitis, when inflammation is present, a low-fiber diet is often recommended to reduce strain on the digestive system and allow the inflamed areas of the colon to heal. However, once the acute phase has passed, gradually reintroducing high-fiber foods into your diet is essential for long-term management and prevention of diverticulitis flare-ups.

Meal Planning and Preparation Tips

1. Embrace High-Fiber Foods: While a low-fiber diet may be necessary during acute episodes, it's crucial to gradually reintroduce fiber-rich foods into your diet once symptoms subside. Incorporate plenty of fruits, vegetables, whole grains, and legumes into your meals to promote regular bowel movements and prevent constipation, which can contribute to diverticulitis flare-ups.

2. Diversify Your Diet: Aim for variety in your meals by including a wide range of high-fiber foods. Experiment with different grains like quinoa, barley, and brown rice, and incorporate a colorful array of fruits and vegetables to ensure you're getting a diverse range of nutrients and fiber.

3. Portion Control: Pay attention to portion sizes, especially when reintroducing high-fiber foods. Start with smaller portions and gradually increase serving sizes as your digestive system adjusts. This approach can help prevent discomfort and bloating associated with sudden increases in fiber intake.

4. Prep Ahead: Spend time each week planning and preparing meals that include high-fiber ingredients. Chop fruits and vegetables, cook whole grains, and portion out legumes to make mealtime easier and more convenient, even during busy days.

5. Stay Hydrated: Alongside increasing fiber intake, it's essential to stay hydrated by drinking plenty of water throughout the day. By absorbing water in the digestive system, fiber helps to maintain regular bowel motions and wards off constipation. Aim for at least eight glasses of water daily, and consider hydrating foods like cucumbers, melons, and citrus fruits.

Stress Management Techniques

1. Practice Relaxation Techniques: Incorporate relaxation techniques such as deep breathing, meditation, or gentle yoga into your daily routine. These practices can help reduce stress levels and promote overall well-being, which is essential for maintaining digestive health.

2. Engage in Physical Activity: Regular exercise is beneficial for both physical and mental health. Find activities you enjoy, such as walking, swimming, or cycling, and aim for at least 30 minutes of moderate exercise most days of the week. Exercise helps reduce stress, improve digestion, and support overall wellness.

3. Prioritize Sleep: Quality sleep is crucial for managing stress and promoting optimal health. Aim for seven to eight hours of uninterrupted sleep each night, and establish a relaxing bedtime routine to help signal to your body that it's time to wind down and prepare for restorative sleep.

4. Seek Support: Don't hesitate to reach out to friends, family, or a support group for emotional support and encouragement. Sharing your experiences with others who understand can provide valuable insight and help alleviate feelings of isolation during challenging times.

5. Set Realistic Goals: Be realistic about what you can accomplish and don't put too much pressure on yourself. Break down huge ambitions into smaller, more doable activities and celebrate your accomplishments along the way. Remember that progress takes time, and be patient with yourself as you navigate your diverticulitis management journey.

Conclusion

As you come to the end of this journey through the Diverticulitis Diet Cookbook, take a moment to reflect on the progress made and the achievements accomplished. Whether you've successfully navigated the acute phase of diverticulitis or implemented long-term dietary changes to manage and prevent flare-ups, each step forward is worth celebrating.

Give yourself credit for the efforts put into adopting healthier eating habits and making positive lifestyle changes. Whether it's incorporating more fiber-rich foods into your diet, mastering meal planning and preparation, or finding effective stress management techniques, every small victory contributes to your overall success in managing diverticulitis.

Moving forward, maintaining healthy eating habits is a lifelong journey. Prioritize nutrient-rich foods, fiber intake, hydration, and stress management to support digestive health and overall well-being. Stay mindful of your body's signals, listen to its needs, and make adjustments as necessary to ensure you're providing it with the nourishment and care it deserves.

In closing, remember you're not alone on this journey. Whether dining out, navigating social gatherings, or facing challenges along the way, you have the knowledge, tools, and support to overcome them and thrive. Keep moving forward with confidence, resilience, and a commitment to your health and happiness.

Scan The QR Code to Get Your Bonus